TABLE OF CONTENTS

W9-BNR-769

ON THE COVER : Eric "Sully" Sullivan finishes the 2010 Ironman St. George with the overall amateur title win. Photo : ASI Photos

Over the last 24 years, we've dramatically improved the performance of tens of thousands of athletes.

Now it's *your* turn.

Fueling, along with training and equipment, are the three critical aspects of endurance athletics. Many athletes focus their time, money, and energy on training and equipment but give only scant attention to fueling. However, shorting your fueling program will put a big dent in the benefit you might have otherwise obtained from hard training and using top-level gear. Why? Because endurance exercise severely stresses your body and depletes your physical reserves. When you fuel your body improperly it's as though you're driving a junker, so to speak, which means that you don't get the full value out of all the time and energy you spent in training. With that being the case, chances are you will never achieve your full potential as an athlete. If athletic achievement is a priority in your life, please heed the information presented in this guide. Learn how to put the right fuels into your body, in the right amounts, at the right time, and you will absolutely reap the benefits—it's a law of nature, and we guarantee it.

Why do so many athletes downplay fueling?

I've often said that there are three key tangibles that are needed to achieve success in athletics:

1. The use of high-quality equipment – You probably don't need the "limited edition, gold plated" model but you do need to use good equipment.

2. The incorporation of an intelligent training and recovery program - You can't just "wing it" in terms of a training regimen and hope that the pieces fall into place. Similarly, you have to recover as "hard" as you train to get the most out of your training.

3. The consistent use of high-quality nutritional supplements and fuels, and a sensible supplement/fueling program.

All three of these tangibles are important and if one is lacking, the others are negatively affected. As mentioned earlier, my sincere belief is that without the consistent use of an intelligent supplement and fueling program, all of the equipment that you spend so much money on and all of the time you spend in training will never realize their full value.

It's pretty easy to get numbers one and two dialed in – the use of high-quality equipment and an intelligent workout/recovery regimen. Number three, especially the fueling component, usually causes so much confusion amongst endurance athletes that they either neglect it entirely or downplay it dramatically.

The sports nutrition market sure doesn't make it easy—it's glutted with hype, cheap sugar-and-sodium-laden products, inappropriately applied research, and a confusing array of products. In addition, it seems as though every issue of your sports magazine of choice trumpets a new "latest and greatest" fueling strategy—such as pre-race sodium loading—with frightening regularity. Or, even worse, some coaches and coaching organizations keep promoting the same archaic fueling recommendations to their athletes, the kind of information that should have died out a long time ago. (Why? Because it didn't work then and it doesn't work now!)

With all of the misinformation bombarding athletes, and with junk food masquerading as "energy fuels," it's easy to understand why you might get frustrated and give up on the idea of developing a sound fueling program. However, despite all of the negatives, fueling remains both vitally important and not all that hard to dial in—once you get the right information.

Article continues on page 6

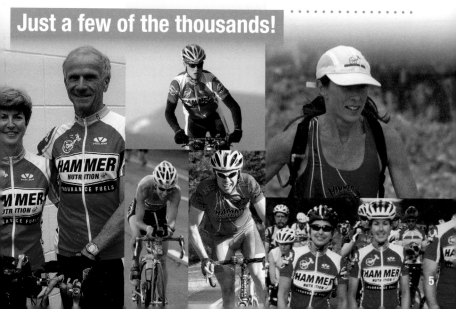

Just a few of the thousands!

Faulty fueling defined

Two analogies will help us understand faulty fueling: a barrel and a gas tank. Imagine a barrel of water with a tap at the bottom. Open the tap and stick a hose in the top of the barrel, filling it at the same rate that the water flows out of the bottom. The input replaces the output. That works fine for a barrel, but our bodies are far more complicated than barrels. The water we drink doesn't go directly to our pores to provide sweat to cool us. Carbohydrates don't go straight down our esophagus to our muscles to provide energy. Instead, we have complex mechanisms that transport, distribute, break down, store, retrieve, and utilize the water and nutrients that we consume. It's impossible just to plug in a hose and resupply at the rate we expend nutrients and water. If we try to refuel thinking that our body is like a barrel, and all we need to do is measure what comes out of the tap and then adjust the input hose accordingly, we'll soon be in big trouble. We'll get oversupplied, disrupt our internal systems, and suffer physiological and performance consequences that range from merely uncomfortable nuisances, like stopping often to pee, to the rare but fatal case of extreme water intoxication.

The second way to picture faulty fueling is the gas tank analogy. Your car has a gas tank that stores enough gas to run the engine for many hours. You can refill in a few minutes and you're set for another several hours of drive time. Some people try to fuel this way, but the human body does not come equipped with an internal fuel tank. We do have some storage capacity, such as muscle glycogen and body fluids, but we can't slug down 500 calories and a liter of water in a few minutes and think that we're good for an hour or more of exercise. Our tanks must be external (e.g., water

The author makes his way through the Mojave Desert during his Double Furnace Creek 508 record attempt in 2002. Photo : Jeff Martin bottles) and we must adjust our consumption to our body's intake capacity. We can only resupply as much as we can process at one time, and that means the right amounts at the right time.

Some personal "learning it the hard way" experiences

In my first Race Across America (RAAM) in 1988, I found out what happens when one ignores the complex physiology of the magnificent organism that is the human body and fuels their body improperly. I learned the hard way that we cannot come anywhere close to replacing the amounts of fluids, calories, and salt/electrolytes that we expend during intense exercise. Like so many athletes then and now, I fueled my body under the belief that since I was losing "X" amount per hour I needed to consume "X", or I'd bonk. What I didn't take into account—and this is the sad truth with so many athletes today—is that the human body knows that it can't effectively replace the full amount of what it loses right away and that it has numerous built-in mechanisms that make up for the shortfall.

Somehow, I did finish the cross-country race, but trust me, I spent most of the time in miserable discomfort. My crew, dutifully following my demands, gorged me with ridiculous amounts of calories and bloated me with excessive fluids. Common sense might have told me to back off, but stubbornness and the mental numbness of round the clock cycling kept me on the same insane regimen. Thinking that I was doing

the right thing, I adhered to my plan for the majority of the race. Stomach distress, bloating, and nausea? This was RAAM, where self-inflicted misery is par for the coast-to-coast course. I felt sick to my stomach most of the time and gained so much water weight (due to my high salt intake) that my belly darn near touched the top tube when I was down on the drops. That's some serious bloating! My inept fueling protocol was the culprit for all of these maladies.

Another example? My lack of knowledge regarding how important protein is during prolonged bouts of exercise and, especially, after exercise. When I first became intrigued by the possible benefits that fuels and supplements might have on my performance and health, I thought I'd check out the local health food store to see what was available. Pretty much what I remember after walking up and down the aisles of the store was that most of what lined the shelves were industrial size containers of protein powders. A good majority of the products I saw had labels that were largely taken up by photos of monstrously huge bodybuilders. A long time passed before I realized that protein isn't just for bodybuilders; it's a necessity for endurance athletes as well.

Speaking of protein, it's a vital component for supporting optimal recovery. Recovery? What's that? Well, for many years my "recovery strategy" after a workout—even a really long, hard workout—was "I'm definitely going to sack out after this one's in the shed." And when the workout was done, that's precisely what I did: I'd hit the shower, then dive on the couch, and not even think about eating anything—let alone a high-quality recovery drink or meal—until much later. I didn't realize it at the time, but I was totally blowing it by not making an effort to "refill the tank," which would have allowed me to get the most out of all the time and energy I spent in the workout.

Here's another example of how I learned to fuel the hard way. I readily admit that throughout the years I've made plenty of mistakes in all aspects of fueling—fluid intake, calorie consumption, and electrolyte replenishment. However, of all the blunders I've made, I'd choose the 1995 Race Across America as my all-time disaster. I was in peak physical condition but I was not prepared for the extreme heat I encountered during the first day through the Mojave Desert. I became dehydrated, was electrolyte depleted, and ended up in the hospital where they reconstituted me with eight liters of IV fluid! My Race Across America never made it across California. Just a few hours of inadequate electrolyte and water intake wiped out months of training, not to mention thousands of dollars. I can laugh about it now ("Hey, I just did the world's most expensive double century") but it sure wasn't a laughing matter back then or for several months afterward.

So you see, I've made lots and lots of mistakes over the years in terms of how to fuel the body prior to, during, and after exercise. In fact, I think I've committed all but one of the mistakes that are listed in the

article "THE TOP 10–The biggest mistakes endurance athletes make" many, many times (and yes, that includes the "honorable mention" as well). The only mistake I didn't make was in regards to pre-exercise fueling. I'd like to say it was because I had an understanding of the rationale behind the recommendations, but in reality I was only doing the right things by accident; I didn't have a clue as to why I was doing what I was doing, even if it was correct.

The reason I bring this up is because all of the mistakes that I've just illustrated are ones that you can avoid . . . and I want you to avoid them! They not only cost me a lot of time, money, and energy, some of them nearly cost me my life!

I've been an endurance athlete for twenty-some years now, and I've been involved with the health food industry equally as long. I've tried just about every pill, powder, and potion out there, only to be disappointed time and again. Trust me, I completely understand the frustration and confusion you may be feeling. Part of my frustration had to do with the poor quality of the products I was testing "back in the day," but I was equally dismayed at the lack of knowledge on how to properly fuel my body in the first place. It took a lot of independent studying and, as I've illustrated in great detail, a lot of trial and error as well ("trial and disaster" might be more accurate).

However, after many years, I eventually learned a lot about proper fueling. The quality of my workouts improved dramatically and with better workouts came increased performance and impressive race results. It took some time, but when I had a good grasp of the key principles, I wanted to share them with endurance athletes around the world. It sounds cliché, I know, but if I can save you some of the headaches and heartaches that I went through, then I've accomplished something major; that's precisely where this book comes in and why it exists.

"The Guide" is born

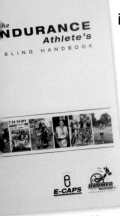

The first Guide, circa 2001

Several years ago two of my colleagues joined me in a project aimed at helping end athletes' confusion. Brian Frank (owner/CEO of Hammer Nutrition), Dr. Bill Misner (who is now retired as Hammer Nutrition's R&D chief), and I wrote and published a little booklet, *The Endurance Athlete's GUIDE to SUCCESS*. Though brief, *The GUIDE* contained a wealth of knowledge culled from our collective six-plus decades and tens of thousands of miles of endurance athletics training. In addition to the latest research (which we, of course, still vigilantly keep up with), the booklet also contained practical information. Our personal experience (much of which was my trial and error "experiments"), in addition to our work with thousands of athletes,

provided us with a unique insight into what works and what doesn't.

Even in its first incarnation, a slender 22 pages, *The GUIDE* had an incredibly positive effect. Finally, endurance athletes had straight talk on the key aspects of athletic fueling. Now in its ninth edition and over 150 pages long, *The GUIDE* has had a total print run of over 100,000 hard copies. That impressive figure, however, pales in comparison to the number of free downloads from the Hammer Nutrition website, which has exceeded one half million! The testimonials we routinely receive clearly indicate that we have filled a very much-needed niche in endurance nutrition. The practical, easy-to-read and easy-to-apply information was guiding—and continues to guide—many athletes to the best performances of their careers.

Our key principle

I'd like to particularly point your attention to the first article, "LESS IS BEST–The right way to fuel." The principle set out in this article is the cornerstone for the entire program, and thus we recommend that you read this article first. The remainder of the articles will have more relevance if set in the context of our basic approach to all fueling. Our detailed recommendations for hydration, calories, and electrolytes almost invariably call for less than the amounts you may be used to. It might seem counter intuitive, but proper fueling strategy does not mean, "replace what you lose," but "replenish what your body can assimilate and utilize." We want you to use only as much as your body can assimilate, and those amounts typically measure far less than what many an "expert" propose. So please read the "LESS IS BEST" article first and that will dial you in to the rest of the advice in *The GUIDE*.

Fueling AND supplementation fueling advice

Although the primary focus in *The Endurance Athlete's GUIDE to SUCCESS* is about how to properly fuel your body, I believe that supplementation plays an important role, not just for enhancing athletic performance but overall health as well.

I've been labeled a "supplement junkie" for longer than I care to remember. I often get teased about how many of them I take, with more than a few people over the years having asked questions such as, "Why do you take so many

supplements? You're eventually going to die someday anyway, so isn't taking all those pills kind of a waste?" Honestly, if I had a nickel for every time I heard that question . . . but I digress. Seriously though, I am a big believer in the consistent use of an intelligently thought out supplement program and my response to my naysayers is usually something to this effect:

• Yes, as much as possible, I try to consume the best diet I can. However, like you and everyone else, I don't eat an ideal diet all the time, or at least as much as I should (such as when I travel).

• No matter how well I eat, no matter how high quality my diet may be, the nutrient density in the foods I consume won't meet my body's requirements, especially when I'm training and/or stressed from work/personal obligations.

• Along with diet, exercise, stress management, spirituality, and other components, I believe that

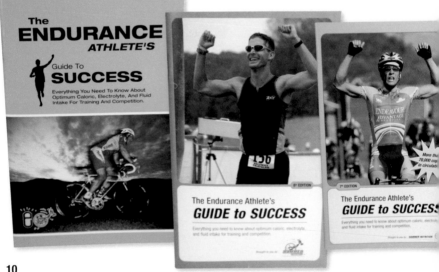

supplementation contributes significantly to my overall well being, so that I can achieve the healthiest, most productive life possible.

• Sure, I'm going to die some day, but I want to postpone that day for as long as possible. Also, when I reach old age, I still want to be mentally and physically active. When I hit my 60's, 70's, and beyond, I don't want to be incapacitated by sickness or disease; I still want to be able to ride my bike, go skiing, and do other activities, and I definitely want my mental faculties intact as well. I don't want to just exist when I get older; I want to live!

These are the primary reasons why I've been an admitted supplement junkie for all of these years. Sure, I've made some mistakes over the years in my supplement purchases (I've wasted a lot of money on supplements that over-promised and greatly under-delivered), but I remain a firm believer that, in addition to a high quality diet, the consistent use of the right supplements has and will continue to pay significant and noticeable benefits. As a result, I have absolutely no regrets and offer no apologies for the amount of supplements I've taken and will continue to take.

So in addition to getting your fueling dialed in—which *The GUIDE* will undoubtedly help with—I hope you will give serious consideration to incorporating an intelligent supplement program in your daily routine. It really can pay some significant dividends when it comes to both your athletic performance and your overall health. We've got some really great information to share with you on this topic and you'll find these articles in the supplement to this book. *The Hammer Nutrition Fuels & Supplements–Everything you need to know.*

Get ready to succeed!

If you're reading this book, you're probably committed to achieving op-timal performance in your training and racing. For over 24 years we've held an unwavering commitment to helping athletes do just that. That's why we're extremely gratified that we have now published our ninth edition of *The GUIDE*, and that this copy is in your hands. If you apply the information in these pages, we guarantee you'll be pleased with the results.

Steve Born
Fueling Expert

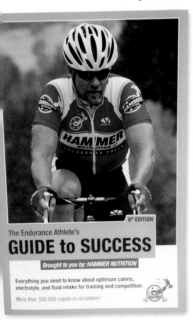

8ᵗʰ EDITION

The Endurance Athlete's
GUIDE to SUCCESS

Brought to you by: HAMMER NUTRITION

Everything you need to know about optimum caloric, electrolyte, and fluid intake for training and competition.

More than 500,000 copies in circulation!

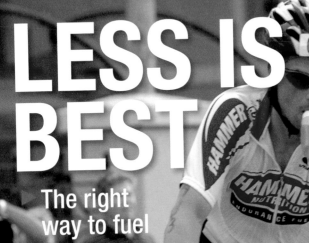

LESS IS BEST

The right way to fuel

Frankie McDermond multitasks at the St. Anthony's Tri in St. Petersburg, Florida.
Photo : ASI Photos

Replenishment vs. replacement

1. This general article states our fundamental approach towards fueling during exercise, which holds true for calorie, water, and electrolyte intake. **The key words are in the title: we cannot replace everything that we expend during exercise, but we can keep ourselves going all day long if we replenish appropriately.**

2. Replenishment means supplying what our bodies can actually absorb and utilize. Using absorption/utilization parameters rather than the expenditure parameter gives us realistic amounts to guide our refueling. **When it comes to fueling, more is not better; smarter is better. Know your body's capacities and ignore the "expenditure" hype.**

3. Not only is the ignorance-based "replace your entire expenditure" strategy (e.g., 800 cal/hr) physiologically unsound, it is costly and unnecessary. **Replacement-guided fueling strategies fail to take into account the obvious fact that our body is a tremendous storehouse of nutrients.**

4. Less obvious, but **equally important, is the fact that our complex physiological pathways negate the idea of simple "calories out/calories in" accounting.** The same holds true for water, electrolytes, or anything else.

5. Using the replacement fueling strategy, an athlete can over-consume up to three, or even four, times what his or her body can actually deal with during exercise. **As a rule of thumb, calorie/water/electrolyte intake will run approximately one-third of expenditure during endurance exercise.**

6. **Over-consumption maladies include a variety of GI and muscle system problems that will cause much distress,** impair performance, and probably leave you far behind the wisely-fueling athletes in the Hammer Nutrition logo clothing.

Start reading the full article on page 14

INTRODUCTION

This is the keynote article on what constitutes proper fluid, calorie, and electrolyte intake during exercise. Our scientifically and experientially established position is this: replenish your body with what it can comfortably accept instead of trying to replace what your body expends. You must calculate your fluid, calorie, and electrolyte intake in accord with your body's absorption mechanisms, not according to its output. If you follow this principle, you will greatly reduce or entirely avoid bloating, cramping, nausea, vomiting, diarrhea, and bonking. Fueling your body in a way that works with it, instead of against it, not only feels better, it also yields higher quality workouts and improved race results.

Your body is extraordinarily designed and knows how to regulate itself when it comes to fueling. During prolonged exercise, it does need your help, but you must cooperate with your body's innate survival mechanisms. Give your body "a helping hand" by providing it with what it can effectively assimilate (instead of trying to replace everything it's losing), and I absolutely guarantee that you will feel better during exercise and enjoy dramatic performance improvements.

FULL ARTICLE

At Hammer Nutrition, we consistently deal with many fueling myths, and I'd rate the "replace what you lose" approach as probably the worst offender of all. Many organizations and alleged experts continue to recommend that athletes need to replace what they expend during exercise in equal or near-equal amounts, hour after hour. They cite data such as "you lose up to two grams of sodium per hour, burn up to 900 calories hourly, and sweat up to two liters an hour" to defend their position. Even worse, sometimes they don't give any numeric guidelines, just vague statements like "take salt tablets" or "drink as much as you can." Sadly, far too many athletes fuel their bodies exactly this way and they get only poorer-than-expected results or a DNF to show for their efforts.

The figures that the "replacement" proponents cite are often valid: a vigorously exercising athlete, especially a big guy, can really expend significant amounts of fluids, calories, and sodium. We don't argue at all with most expenditure figures. However, expenditure just isn't the appropriate measure to guide your fueling, it is what you can effectively assimilate. Don't go by what you burn/lose, but rather what the body can reasonably absorb and process during any given period of time.

The statements on page 15 from Dr. Bill Misner represent our position on what proper fueling is all about.

What this means is that the body cannot replace fluids and nutrients at the same rate it depletes them.

Article continues on page 16

Thoughts on proper fueling

"To suggest that fluids, sodium, and fuels-induced glycogen replenishment can happen at the same rate as it is spent during exercise is simply not true. Endurance exercise beyond 1-2 hours is a deficit spending entity, with proportionate return or replenishment always in arrears. The endurance exercise outcome is to postpone fatigue, not to replace all of the fuel, fluids, and electrolytes lost during the event. It can't be done, though many of us have tried."

"The human body has so many survival safeguards by which it regulates living one more minute, that when we try too hard to fulfill all of its needs we interfere, doing more harm than good."

- William Misner, Ph.D. - Director of Research & Product Development, Emeritus

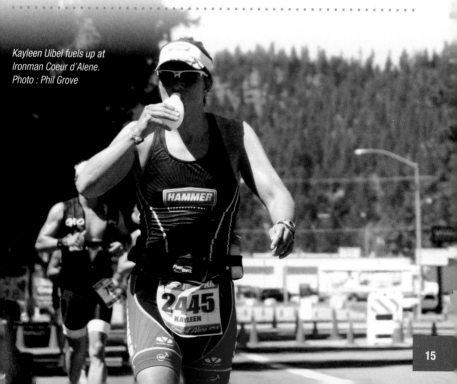

Kayleen Uibel fuels up at Ironman Coeur d'Alene.
Photo : Phil Grove

The Fast Lane

▶ For calories, on average, only 30-40% of what is utilized ("burned") can be efficiently replenished. In general, fluids are replenished at a rate of only 20-33% of what is spent, and sodium 20-35%.

▶ If you err on the "not enough" side in regards to calories, that's a very easy problem to fix—you simply consume more calories. However, if you over-supply your body with too many calories, that's a much harder (and longer) problem to resolve (at the very least you'll have to deal with an upset stomach for quite awhile).

▶ Body fat stores satisfy upwards of two-thirds of energy requirements, very easily making up the difference between what is burned and what the body can accept in replenishment.

Article continues here

Yes, the body needs your assistance in replenishing what it loses, but that donation must be in amounts that cooperate with normal body mechanisms, not in amounts that override them. Here's an important fact to keep in mind: at an easy aerobic pace, the metabolic rate increases 1200-2000% over the sedentary state. As a result, the body goes into "survival mode," where blood volume is routed to working muscles, fluids are used for evaporative cooling mechanisms, and oxygen is routed to the brain, heart, and other internal organisms. With all of this going on, your body isn't terribly interested in handling large quantities of calories, fluids, and electrolytes; its priorities lie elsewhere.

Your body already "knows" it is unable to immediately replenish calories, fluids, and electrolytes at the same rate it uses/loses them, and it has the ability to effectively deal with this issue. That's why we don't recommend trying to replace hourly losses of calories, fluids, and electrolytes with loss amounts. Instead, we recommend smaller replenishment amounts that cooperate with normal body mechanisms. We'll discuss this in more detail later in the article.

What does research show regarding replenishment?

The 'Loss vs. Assimilation' table on page 17 is a suggested comparison showing approximated upper values for what is lost during prolonged endurance exercise to the maximal amount that can be successfully absorbed, replaced, and routed into the energy cycle for the average-size endurance athlete (160-165 lbs/72.5-75 kg) who is fit and acclimatized.

As you can see, there is a tremendous difference between what is lost and what can effectively be replenished during exercise. For calories, on average only 30-

Loss vs. Assimilation
What can your body really handle?

SUBSTANCE	RATE LOSS/hr	ASSIMILATION RATE
Fluids (ml)	1000-3000 (30-90 oz)	500-830 (17-28 oz)
Sodium (mg)	2000	500-700
Calories	700-900	240-280

Below are the corresponding replenishment values that we have observed for the average-size endurance athlete (160-165 lbs/72.5-75 kg) who is fit and acclimatized (+/-5%):

SUBSTANCE	IDEAL REPLENISHMENT
Fluids	20-33%
Sodium	20-35%
Fuels (Calories)	30-40%

References:
• Noakes T.D., 2003, Lore of Running. Leisure Press. Champaign Illinois. Pages 768-770 29 published and unpublished papers cited on fuels, fluids, electrolyte issues during endurance exercise.
• Moodley D. et al., 1992, Exogenous carbohydrate oxidation during prolonged exercise. The effect of carbohydrate type and solution concentration. Unpublished manuscript in #1 above.
• Sweat Composition in Exercise and Heat. Verde T, Shephard RJ, Corey P, Moore R, 1982, J Appl Phys 53(6) 1541-1542.
• Sweating: Its composition and effects on body fluids. Costill DL, 1977 & 1982, Annals of the New York Academy of Sciences, 301, p.162.
• American Dietetics Association Position Statement
• American College of Sports Medicine Position Statement

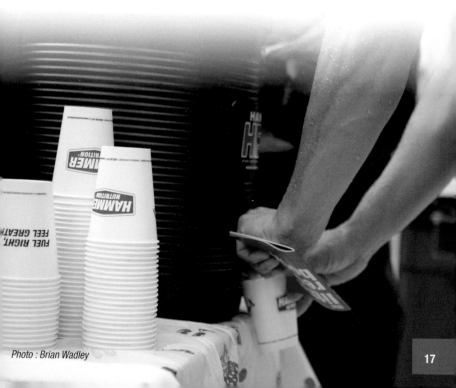

Photo : Brian Wadley

The Fast Lane

▶ The safe rule of thumb is to replenish at about one-third of loss values, obviously adjusting as conditions dictate.

▶ Your body already "knows" it is unable to immediately replenish calories, fluids, and electrolytes at the same rate it uses/loses them, and it has the ability to effectively deal with this issue. That's why we don't recommend trying to replace hourly losses of calories, fluids, and electrolytes with loss amounts. Instead, we recommend smaller replenishment amounts that cooperate with normal body mechanisms.

▶ The body has remarkably complex and efficient "built-in" survival safeguards that very capably deal with the difference between what it loses and what it can accept in replenishment.

Article continues here

40% of what is utilized ("burned") can be efficiently replenished. In general, fluids are replenished at a rate of only 20-33% of what is spent, and sodium 20-35%. What's important to keep in mind is that the body is keenly sensitive to this, recognizing its inability to replenish what it loses at anywhere near the rate that it's losing it.

For example, body fat stores satisfy upwards of two-thirds of energy requirements, very easily making up the difference between what is burned and what the body can accept in replenishment. For the majority of athletes, calorie oxidation rate and gastric absorption rate typically allow for no more than 280 calories per hour—at the most—to be consumed for successful gastric absorption to energy transfer. Consuming greater than 280 cal/hr increases the potential for a number of stomach/digestive distress issues.

In regards to body fluid volume and serum sodium concentration, both are controlled to a degree by hormone pathways between the brain and internal organs. As Dr. Misner stated, the body has remarkably complex and efficient "built-in" survival safeguards that very capably deal with the difference between what it loses and what it can accept in replenishment. The various systems involved are complex, but the bottom line is that only a relatively small consumption will keep you going. On the other hand, over-consumption can easily throw the systems out of whack.

This is why we are so adamant about the "less is best" way of fueling. For example, if you err on the "not enough" side in regards to calories, that's a very easy problem to fix – you simply consume more calories. However, if you over-supply your body with too many calories, that's a much harder (and longer) problem to resolve (at the very least you'll have to deal with an upset stomach for quite awhile). The simple truth is that once excess amounts of calories, fluids, and/or sodium are

Fueling variability among athletes

There is no "one size fits all"!

The data from athletes who suffered poor performance due to fueling-related problems

• Fluid intake was almost always over 30 fluid ounces (887ml)/hour.

• Body weight at finish was hyper-hydrated with weight gain from 1-2%, or dehydrated at over 3% body weight loss.

• Excess calorie consumption, at or greater than 300 cal/hr, primarily from simple sugared-based fuels, causing stomach shutdown.

• High sodium diets. Athletes who consume this type of diet are predisposed to higher sodium intake during an event than the low sodium purist.

• Ultra distance athletes who suffered cramps, sour stomach, malaise, and/or hyponatremia in the last half of their event often did not train adequately at race-level fluid/fuel/electrolyte dosing, or the athlete used a different fueling protocol than in training. Athletes need to not only train appropriately leading up to their race, they also must test, evaluate, and fine-tune their fueling plan in training prior to using it in a race.

The data from athletes reporting success (no fuel-related, performance-inhibiting problems and consistent energy levels)

• Fluid intake was at or under 28 fluid ounces (828ml)/hour.

• Electrolyte intake via Endurolytes was between 3-6 capsules/hour, with 4 capsules/hour being the most often reported dose.

• Calorie intake was at 280/hour or less.

• Body weight at finish decreased no more than 2-3%.

What you should derive from all of this is that while there is no "one size fits all" fueling formula, there are some good guidelines in terms of what has been shown to be successful for athletes and also consistent observations (read: fueling errors) noted from athletes who had unsuccessful races.

Read our fueling recommendations on the next page

Our fueling recommendations

Based on what science has shown us, plus over two decades of working with athletes, we have determined the following ranges as ideal for most athletes, the majority of the time, for maintaining optimal exercise performance:

Fluids:
16-28 oz/hour

Sodium Chloride:
100-600 mg/hour
(1-6 Endurolytes)

Calories:
150-280/hour

The Fast Lane

▶ Hot weather usually means lower hourly calorie intake, a slightly higher fluid intake, and an increased electrolyte intake.

▶ High impact exercise does better with roughly 30%-50% lower caloric intake per hour than what you'd consume during a less jarring exercise.

▶ Over-supplying your body will absolutely not enhance athletic performance but will most definitely inhibit-or-ruin it.

Article continues here

in your body they're not coming out, at least not the way that you want them to! Bottom line? Over-supplying your body will absolutely not enhance athletic performance but will most definitely inhibit-or-ruin it.

Of course, there are many individual variations that you will need to consider (age, weight, training/racing stress, fitness, acclimatization levels, weather conditions) to determine what works best for you. Some athletes will need less than these suggested amounts, a handful slightly more. Certain circumstances require flexibility; for instance, hot weather and high-impact exercise, such as the run portion of a long-distance triathlon. Hot weather usually means lower hourly calorie intake, a slightly higher fluid intake, and an increased electrolyte intake. High impact exercise such as running does better with roughly 30%-50% lower caloric intake per hour than what you'd consume during a less jarring exercise such as cycling.

All of this said, the figures listed make good starting points for determining your ideal intakes for varying conditions and circumstances. As far as calorie intake is concerned, we highly recommend that you use our weight-specific dosage suggestions, which are listed in the article "THE HAMMER NUTRITION FUELS–What they are and how to use them" in the supplement to this guide.

SUMMARY

Proper fueling is consuming the least amount necessary to keep your body doing what you want it to do hour after hour.

We have been advocating the "less is best" recommendation for over two decades. Sadly, many athletes continue to listen to "consume what you lose" propaganda, arguing that nutrients and water need to be replaced immediately. This is neither true nor possible; fluids, calories, and electrolytes cannot be replaced 100%, or even 50%. As a result of following this flawed advice, athletes continue to experience cramping, vomiting, gastric distress, diarrhea, and other problems. The safe rule of thumb is to replenish at about one-third of loss values, obviously adjusting as conditions dictate.

As you read through our other fueling-related articles, you'll see this principle applied repeatedly and further details given. It might seem like we're banging the same drum all the time, but when it comes to fueling, we cannot emphasize enough that less is better than more. Rather than attempting to resolve your fueling requirements by replacing hourly loss with hourly intake, we suggest small doses, generally about a third of what is lost, if not lower. In conjunction with long-standing research regarding this subject, over two decades of successful experience with athletes testifies to the reliability of the "less is best" and "fuel in cooperation with your body" concepts. Yes, there are people who can complete events on high intakes of fluids, calories, and electrolytes, but the overwhelming majority of athletes are impaired or stopped by such fueling protocols. Athletes who do use less see their fueling-related problems end and their performance improve dramatically.

That's why our battle cry is "Less is Best"! Remember, the goal of fueling is NOT to see how much you can consume and get away with before your body rebels, you end up getting sick, and your performance goes in the tank. Proper fueling is consuming the least amount necessary to keep your body doing what you want it to do hour after hour. And if you do err on the "not enough" side, that's a much easier problem to resolve than an "uh oh, I overdid it" problem. We're pretty darn sure that once you get away from those 500-700 calorie and liter-of-fluid-an-hour regimens, your body will perform much better, you'll feel better, and you'll get the results you trained so hard for.

HYDRATION

► **What you need to know**

Mickey Franco of the Chicago Lions Rugby
Sevens team stays hydrated (and fueled)
by drinking water mixed with Perpetuem.
Photo : Aaron Manheimer

Proper hydration is critical

1. Even though it has no nutrient value, **water is the most critical of all your exercise fueling needs.**

2. It is, of course, vital to drink water and prevent dehydration; however, **excess water intake is probably more common and causes worse problems.**

3. **Excess water consumption is especially common among inexperienced and "back-of-the-pack" athletes.** These athletes are prone to a variety of discomforts such as bloating, frequent urination, the effects of electrolyte depletion, and in extreme cases, water intoxication, which can be lethal.

4. **Dehydration most likely occurs in front-running and highly competitive athletes who don't take the time to properly hydrate or who overestimate their** "toughness." Dehydration will severely impair performance and can easily buy you a DNF and an IV; not the letters you want!

5. **For most athletes, the majority of the time, an intake of roughly one water bottle per hour (approx. 20-25 oz) will serve you well.** Lighter weight athletes may not need that much, while some larger athletes on a hot day might need to go higher.

6. **If you end a long race or training session with up to a 2% weight loss, you're okay;** more than 3% and you're into noticeable dehydration. No loss, or worse yet, weight gain, would indicate over-hydration.

Start reading the full article on page 24

INTRODUCTION

Water is the most important substance on earth, 60% of your body weight, and the number one concern on any athlete's intake list. For both performance and health, the importance of your water intake exceeds that of your vitamin, calorie, and electrolyte consumption. We want to make sure that you have the right amount on board when you set off on your distance efforts, when you finish, and between efforts during recovery; hence the inclusion of this article in *The GUIDE*. You'll learn how sweat loss affects athletic performance, that too much water is as bad, if not worse, than too little, and that you can't replace all of the water that you sweat out. Yes, we will get to the key issue: Just how much should I drink? Of all the many functions water has in human physiology, we'll focus on just a couple that pertain especially to the endurance athlete: cooling the body and transporting nutrients. Let's look at the cooling system first.

FULL ARTICLE

When we exercise, we burn molecular fuel (mostly glycogen) but also some protein, fat, and blood glucose from ingested nutrients. The breakdown of these energy providers releases heat that builds up and raises our core temperature. The body must rid itself of this heat and maintain a core temperature within a few degrees of the well-known 98.6° F (37° C). An active person needs a reliable cooling mechanism. Actually, you have several. You lose some heat through your skin. Blood carries heat to the capillaries near the skin's surface, removing heat from the body core. You breathe harder to get more oxygen, expelling heat when you exhale. But by far the most important part of the cooling system, accounting on average for about 75% of all cooling, is your ability to produce and excrete sweat.

Sweat, however, glistening on your forearm or soaking your singlet won't cool you; it must evaporate. Sweat works on a basic physical premise: water evaporation is an endothermic process, requiring energy (heat) to change from liquid to gas. Thus, water molecules in the gas phase have more energy than water molecules in the liquid phase. As water molecules evaporate from your skin, they remove heat energy; the remaining water molecules have less energy and you feel cooler. Isn't that cool?

Weather conditions greatly affect sweat production and cooling effectiveness. In cool weather, you get substantial cooling from the heat that escapes directly from your skin. As the temperature increases, you gradually rely more on evaporation. On hot days, with little difference between skin surface and ambient temperatures, your skin surface provides only negligible convective cooling, and you need to sweat more to maintain a safe internal core temperature. At 95° F (35° C) or above, you lose no heat at all from your skin; in fact, you actually start to absorb heat. Evaporative cooling must do all of the work.

Humidity is the other major factor that affects sweat. On humid days, sweat evaporates more slowly because the atmosphere is already saturated with water vapor, retarding the evaporation rate. The sweat accumulates on your skin and soaks your clothes, but you don't get any cooling from it because it's not going into the vapor phase. Soaking, dripping sweat may give you a psychological boost, but it has no physical efficacy to cool; sweat must evaporate to remove heat. On days when it's both hot and humid, well, you don't need to read about what's going to happen when you exercise in those conditions. You do need to know that under the worst of conditions you can produce up to three liters of sweat in an hour of strenuous exercise, but your body can only absorb about one liter from fluid consumption. Yes, this will cause problems before long, and we will discuss that issue below.

What happens when the coolant runs low?

Just like a car, your body must dissipate the excess heat generated from burning fuel. Unlike a car, your body's coolant isn't in a sealed internal system; you use it once and then it's gone and needs to be replaced. Unfortunately, we don't come with built-in gauges or indicators that tell us just how much coolant we have left in our system. We can't run a dipstick down our gullet and get a reading that says, "Add a quart." We do have some physiological signs, but they

function at the "Warning-Danger!" level, too late to maintain optimal performance. For instance, by the time you feel thirsty, you could have a 2% body weight water loss, already into the impairment zone.

The chart on page 27 shows what happens to human performance at each percent of weight loss. By weight loss, we mean the percentage of your body weight at the start of exercise that you have lost at the end via sweat. If you go out for a run at 160 pounds (approx 72.5 kg) and weigh in 20 miles later at 154 (approx 70 kg), you've lost almost 4% of your body weight. That's too much to maintain your pace to the end, let alone expect to kick.

. . . .

Humidity is the other major factor that affects sweat. On humid days, sweat evaporates more slowly because the atmosphere is already saturated with water vapor, retarding the evaporation rate. The sweat accumulates on your skin and soaks your clothes, but you don't get any cooling from it because it's not going into the vapor phase.

. . . .

How much is that?

As you can see from the chart on page 27, sweat loss can easily escalate from an athletic performance issue to an acute medical issue. Clearly, we need to have some quantifiable idea of our intake and output. Let's start with converting the data on the

▶ One pint = one water
bottle. Some bottles hold
20 ounces (approx 590 ml),
but consider a regular water
bottle as a pint (16 ounces/
approx 475 ml).

Two pints make a quart (32
ounces), which is equivalent
to almost a liter – not quite,
but almost. So when you
read "liter," think two water
bottles. Losing one pound
of weight means a one-pint
loss. One liter (or one quart)
is about two pounds.

▶ On average, you lose about
one liter (about 34 ounces)
of fluid per hour of exercise.
Extreme heat and humidity
can raise that amount to
three liters in one hour.

✳ Article Reference
"LESS IS BEST–The
right way to fuel"
Page 12

chart to recognizable amounts. Perhaps you
remember the saying, "a pint's a pound,
the world 'round." Now that's a convenient
conversion for endurance athletes. Here's
another: one pint = one water bottle. Some
bottles hold 20 ounces (approx 590 ml), but
consider a regular water bottle as a pint
(16 ounces/approx 475 ml). Two pints make
a quart (32 ounces), which is equivalent
to almost a liter—not quite, but almost.
So when you read "liter," think two water
bottles. Losing one pound of weight (slightly
less than half a kilogram) means a one-pint
loss. One liter (or one quart) is about two
pounds (nearly one kilogram).

Can you drink enough?

Needless to say, maintaining optimal fluid
intake prior to and during exercise is crucial
for both performance and health. However,
as is true with calories and electrolytes,
you can't replenish fluids at the same rate
you deplete them; your body simply won't
absorb as fast as it loses. Evaporative cooling
depletes fluids and electrolytes faster than
the body can replenish them. Your body will
accept and utilize a certain amount from
exogenous (outside) sources, and, similar to
calories and electrolytes, maintaining fluid
intake within a specific range will postpone
fatigue and promote peak performance.

Research suggests that while electrolyte
needs for individual athletes may vary up
to 1000% (tenfold), fluid loss remains fairly
constant. Also, we can measure fluid loss
more easily than electrolyte loss; we don't
need sophisticated lab equipment, just a
scale. Thus, we can come pretty close in
calculating fluid loss and replacement.

The numbers

On average, you lose about one liter (approx
34 ounces) of fluid per hour of exercise.
Extreme heat and humidity can raise that
amount to three liters in one hour. A trained

Symptoms by percent body weight water loss

0% None, optimal performance, normal heat regulation

1% Thirst stimulated, heat regulation during exercise altered, performance declines

2% Further decrease in heat regulation, hinders performance, increased thirst

3% More of the same (worsening performance)

4% Exercise performance cut by 20 - 30%

5% Headache, irritability, "spaced-out" feeling, fatigue

6% Weakness, severe loss of thermoregulation

7% Collapse likely unless exercise stops

8+% Detrimental to health

Nutrition for Cyclists, Grandjean & Ruud, Clinics in Sports Med. Vol 13(1);235-246. Jan 1994

. . . .

Article continues here

athlete will store enough muscle glycogen to provide energy for approximately 90 minutes of aerobic exercise. As your muscles burn glycogen, water is released as a metabolic by-product and excreted as sweat. Researchers found that during a marathon (26.2 miles), runners released an average of two liters of sweat from muscle glycogen stores. This is in addition to sweat from other body liquids.

You can control or lessen these sweat rates by acclimatization and training for the event. Acclimatized athletes can reduce electrolyte and fluid loss up to 50%, but note that those losses cannot be fully replaced during the event. Remember the words of Dr. Bill Misner (mentioned in the "LESS IS BEST–The right way to fuel"* article), "The endurance exercise

The Fast Lane

▶ A trained athlete will store enough muscle glycogen to provide energy for approximately 90 minutes of aerobic exercise.

▶ Use caffeine with caution. Used properly and sparingly, caffeine has ergogenic benefits. It does, however, act as a diuretic, which may deplete fluid stores more rapidly.

▶ Urine color can indicate hydration level. Dark yellow urine means low hydration. Pale to light yellow is good. Don't confuse the bright yellow urine you get after vitamin B-2 (riboflavin) supplementation for the dark yellow urine that indicates overly concentrated urine.

outcome is to postpone fatigue, not replace all the fuel, fluids, and electrolytes lost during the event. It can't be done, though many of us have tried." In other words, our hydration goal is not to replace water ounce-for-ounce or pint-for-pint, but to support natural stores by consuming as much as we can adequately process during exercise.

At the most, you can absorb about one liter (approx 34 fluid ounces) of water per hour, but only in the most extreme heat and humidity. Most of the time you can only absorb about half or not too much over half that amount, even though it won't fully replace your losses. Repeated intake of one liter (about 34 fluid ounces) per hour will ultimately do you more harm than good.

Can you drink too much?

Ironically, while you can't drink enough to replace all fluid lost, you can drink too much. Researchers have noted the dangers of excess hydration during events lasting over four hours. Dr. Tim Noakes collected data for ten years from some 10,000 runners participating in the Comrades Marathon. This 52.4-mile (84.33 km) race, held each June (winter) in South Africa, ranks as one of the world's premier ultra marathons. Noakes showed that endurance athletes who consumed from 16-24 fluid ounces per hour (approx 475-710 milliliters) typically replenished as much fluid as is efficiently possible. He also noted the prevalence of hyponatremia (low blood sodium) during ultra marathons and triathlons in runners who hydrated excessively. This condition can arise from several different physiological scenarios. For endurance athletes, it usually results from sweat-depleted sodium stores diluted by excess hypotonic (low electrolyte content) fluid intake. When blood sodium concentration becomes too dilute, you can develop severe cardiac symptoms leading to collapse.

Problems with too much or too little

Moreover, Noakes noted a pattern of hydration problems among race participants. In ultra events, the leaders usually dehydrate, but the athletes in the middle-to-back of the pack tend to overhydrate. Both may end up suffering from the same hyponatremic symptoms; the former from too little fluid intake combined with too much sodium loss due to profuse sweating, the latter from too much fluid intake and relatively less sodium loss. Because most front-runners are extremely competitive, they don't stop long enough during the race to overhydrate. In addition, it's highly likely that elite athletes may be fitter and better acclimatized to deal with hot weather conditions. A tendency to linger at aid stations, attempting to relieve the symptoms of fatigue or heat by drinking too much water, is a fault found among the majority of the remainder of athletes, those in the middle

or back of the pack. Also, these athletes may be novices who have heard the "drink, drink, drink" mantra, but who haven't had enough experience to personally calibrate their individual needs. After the 1985 Comrades race, 17 runners were hospitalized, nine with dilutional hyponatremia. In the 1987 Comrades Marathon, 24 runners suffered from dilutional hyponatremia. These athletes had seriously overloaded on fluid intake, with the inevitable result of a totally disrupted physiology.

Tragic consequences

Hyponatremia usually results from drinking too much, especially when one drinks fluids such as plain water or a sports drink lacking the proper electrolyte profile. Training and fitness levels, weather conditions, and, undoubtedly, biological predisposition also contribute to developing this form of hyponatremia known as "water intoxication."

The Fast Lane

▶ Don't assume that you can drink unlimited amounts of water or fluid during exercise and expect that all of it will be absorbed and the excess will be lost in sweat or through the kidneys. You will instead bloat, dilute your blood, urinate excessively, and develop water intoxication.

▶ Use cold fluids as much as possible as your body absorbs them more rapidly than warm fluids. Know where to find cold water along your training routes. Use frozen and insulated water bottles and hydration packs.

* Article Reference
"THE TOP 10—The biggest mistakes endurance athletes make"
Page 106

Sadly, we must note that this condition has led, directly or in part, to the deaths of otherwise healthy runners in major American marathons. It is hard for us to comprehend the grief of the families they left behind. These athletes went out to run a marathon, to achieve a personal victory. Improper hydration took away their day of glory and also their lives. They collapsed and went into an irreversible condition involving uncontrollable brain edema, coma, and death. We report this to help prevent any future such tragedies. Overhydration represents a very serious problem. Unlike dehydration, which will generally only result in painful cramping, possibly a DNF, or at the worst, IV treatment, overhydration can incite a chain of ultimately fatal physiological consequences.

So how much, how often?

The extreme cases cited above happen very rarely. Lesser degrees of impairment occur frequently from excessive fluid intake. We don't have a chart for overhydration similar to the one for dehydration. Also, you probably don't carry a scale or have regular access to weigh-ins along your training route. So how do you know when it's time to drink? You don't wait until you're down a quart. A good hydration regimen starts before you even get moving.

Noakes believes intake of hypotonic fluids of one liter/hr (33.8 oz/hr) will likely cause water intoxication and dilutional hyponatremia. He suggests that athletes may do better on 500 ml/hr (approx 17 oz/hr) fluid intake for ultra events performed in hot weather conditions. In "THE TOP 10–The biggest mistakes endurance athletes make"* article, Dr. Ian Rogers suggests that between 500-750 ml/hr (about 17-25 oz/hr) will fulfill most athletes' hydration requirements under most conditions. According to Dr. Rogers, "Like most things in life, balance is

How much fluid should you drink?

Based on the available research, along with the thousands of athletes we have monitored, we have found the following fluid intake amounts to be most beneficial.

Average athlete, average temps

20-25 oz/hr (approx 590-740 ml/hr) is an appropriate fluid intake for most athletes under most conditions.

Lighter athletes or cooler temps

For lighter weight athletes, or those exercising in cooler temperatures, 16-18 oz/hr (approx 473-532 ml) may be perfect.

Heavier athletes or hotter temps

Heavier athletes or athletes competing in hotter conditions may consider intakes upwards of 28 oz/hr (approx 830 ml/hr).

DON'T DRINK TOO MUCH!

We also suggest that to avoid dilutional hyponatremia, fluid intake should not routinely exceed 28 oz/hr (830 ml/hr). The exceptions are heavier athletes, athletes exercising at extreme levels (prolonged periods at a high percentage of VO2Max), and athletes competing in severe environmental conditions.

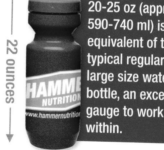

22 ounces

20-25 oz (approx 590-740 ml) is the equivalent of the typical regular-to-large size water bottle, an excellent gauge to work within.

Article continues here

the key and the balance is likely to be at a fluid intake not much above 500 milliliters (about 17 ounces) per hour in most situations, unless predicted losses are very substantial." Other research suggests a similar consumption of 4.5-7.0 oz (approx 133-207 ml) of water every 15 to 20 minutes of exercise.

Remember your electrolytes and calories!

We noted at the beginning of this article that besides cooling, water also plays an important role in nutrient transport. Water consumption bears directly on electrolyte and caloric uptake. You must consider the electrolyte

▶ Train to get fit in the heat. Heat acclimatization and fitness reduce fluid and electrolyte losses by up to 50%.

▶ Know the symptoms of overhydration and dehydration. Stop immediately if you feel lightheaded or queasy or get the dry chills. No race or training is worth compromising your health.

▶ Wear the lightest, most evaporation-friendly clothing you can afford. Cotton isn't on the list. Many fibers today provide superior wicking and evaporation that allow your sweat to do the work nature intended.

✳ Article Reference "ELECTROLYTE REPLENISHMENT–Why it's so important and how to do it right." Page 38

✳ Article Reference "PROPER FUELING– Pre-workout & race suggestions" Page 96

content of your fluid intake, especially if you exceed about 24 oz/hr (710 ml/hr). If temperature and humidity rise above 70° F (21° C) and/or 70% humidity, we recommend that you take electrolytes before and during every hour of exercise. For a full discussion of electrolyte needs, see the article "ELECTROLYTE REPLENISHMENT–Why it's so important and how to do it right."✳

In addition, avoid fructose or other simple sugar-based drinks and gels, especially in the heat – unless you want to deal with a gastric emptying problem, which may result in nausea and other stomach maladies. Compared to complex carbohydrates, drinks or gels that contain simple sugars (typically glucose, fructose, and sucrose) require more fluid and electrolytes for effective absorption. Because they require more fluid, you get fewer calories per unit of water. You must restrict simple sugar drinks to a 6-8% solution range, which provides inadequate amounts of calories for energy production. You can make a nice drink in a water bottle that will absorb well and provide adequate fluid, but your caloric intake will fall far short of your body's needs and your energy level will suffer.

If you make a double or triple-strength batch of a simple sugar drink hoping to obtain adequate amounts of calories, you'll require additional fluids and electrolytes to efficiently process the sugar. You will need to guess how much extra water and electrolytes your body needs to handle the sugar. If you guess low, your GI tract will be forced to pull minerals and fluids from other areas of the body. This scenario can cause nauseating results as your body literally dehydrates its working muscles while bloating your belly. Why take chances like that when your performance is on the line?

Your wisest choice is to use fuel comprised of complex carbohydrates, which is the carbohydrate source of all the Hammer Nutrition fuels. Even at a 15-18%

concentration, these fuel sources absorb and digest rapidly, do not require excess fluid for transport through the GI system, and provide all of the calories your liver can process. For more details on fueling, see the article "PROPER FUELING–Pre-workout & race suggestions"*

Multi-hour bottles of fuel – A convenient way to monitor fluid and calorie intake

If you're going to be exercising for several hours, a convenient and time-efficient way to fuel (while also helping you monitor calorie and fluid intake with greater precision) is to make concentrated, multi-hour bottles of Sustained Energy or Perpetuem. This is discussed in the article "The Hammer Nutrition Fuels" found in the supplement to this book. However, since the topic here is hydration, presenting this information now is relevant.

Each scoop of Sustained Energy and Perpetuem that you put in a bottle reduces the water volume by about 1.5 ounces (approx 44 ml). For example, if you add two scoops of Perpetuem to a 21-ounce (approx 620 ml) water bottle, you won't end up with that same amount of actual fluid; it will be approximately 18 oz (roughly 502 ml), perhaps even slightly less. For some athletes, 18 oz/hr is sufficient, but for many athletes that's not enough; oftentimes upwards of 25-28 oz (approx 740-830 ml) of fluid are required hourly. As a result, you'll have to drink your entire fuel bottle plus plain water from another source. After awhile it can be difficult to keep precise track of your fluid intake because you're fulfilling your needs from two separate sources.

To make things easier when doing a three-hour or longer workout, we suggest making concentrated,

Jamie Donaldson runs up Mt. Evans on a 28-mile training day. Photo : Bob MacGillivray

▶ For your regular daily hydration needs (that is, in addition to your exercise-induced needs), no research has conclusively arrived at an RDA for fluids, but about 0.5-0.6 fluid ounces per pound of body weight (roughly 33-39 ml/kg) makes a more accurate standard than the "eight glasses a day" commonly recommended for everyone. Multiplying your body weight in pounds by 0.5-0.6 will give you the figure, in fluid ounces, that you should aim for daily.

▶ During exercise, avoid foods and fuels that contain short-chain carbohydrates. These simple sugar fuels require more fluids and electrolytes for digestive purposes. Also avoid carbonated drinks, as the gas inhibits absorption.

multi-hour bottles of fuel. For example, if you're going to be exercising for four hours and you know that you need two scoops of Perpetuem to satisfy an hour's worth of fueling, make an 8-scoop bottle in a 21-ounce (approx 620 ml) water bottle. Now you have four hours of fuel in one bottle and that provides a number of benefits:

• Because you have four hours of fuel in one bottle, you only need to drink one-fourth of that bottle hourly, which means you don't have to drink a full bottle of flavored liquid hour after hour.

• You don't need to stop every hour to make more fuel because you've got four hours in one bottle.

• You can drink and enjoy plain water from another source (another bottle, hydration system) to cleanse the palate and satisfy hydration needs.

Yes, there is some actual fluid left in that 8-scoop/4-hour bottle of Perpetuem, but the amount is small, yielding less than four ounces (approx 118 ml) hourly over the course of four hours. Does that small amount of fluid "count" towards fulfilling your overall hydration needs? Yes, but it's a small enough amount to not have to think about if you're keeping your overall fluid intake within our suggested guidelines (approximately 20-25 oz / 590-740 ml hourly). Plus, those hourly guidelines do have some flexibility built in (+/− 3-4 oz or approx 89-118 ml).

With that in mind, a concentrated bottle of Perpetuem can thus be thought of as a "calories only" bottle and you'll fulfill your hydration needs with plain water from another source. The beauty of this, among the other benefits mentioned earlier, is that because you're fulfilling your calorie and fluid needs from sources independent of each other, you're able to gauge your intake with greater precision.

Beat the heat!
Tips to keep cool

▶ A cold, wet towel, sponge, hose, or sprayer on the head and torso.

▶ If you're running, take a one-minute walk, douse yourself with water, and take a good drink.

▶ If you're cycling, find a spot for a good coast or easy spin for a minute. The break from heavy exertion allows dissipation of internal heat.

Combined with hydration and external water, these ideas can effectively relieve heat stress, allowing you to finish hot weather endurance events. Highly competitive athletes might scoff at walking, but when it comes to core temperature, nature gives you two choices: cool down or DNF.

Amanda Carey. Photo : Paul Henry

Article continues here

So when your workouts are greater than three hours in length, give the multi-hour bottle of Sustained Energy or Perpetuem a try and you'll find that it'll be a lot easier to keep track of both your calorie and fluid intake . . . it's been a winning strategy for thousands of endurance athletes.

Fluid intake suggestions apart from the workout or race

Now that you have a good guide for your fluid intake during exercise, we can turn to two other considerations: how much you should drink overall during the day and how you should hydrate just prior to racing or exercise. For your regular daily hydration needs (that is, in addition to your exercise-induced needs), no research has conclusively arrived at an RDA for fluids, but about 0.5-0.6 fluid ounces per pound of body weight (roughly 33-39 ml/kg) makes a more accurate standard than the "eight glasses a day" commonly recommended for everyone. Multiplying your body weight in pounds by 0.5-0.6 will give you the figure, in fluid

▶ If you finish an event weighing the same or more than when you started, you have overhydrated. If you've dropped 3% or more, dehydration has occurred. Up to 2% weight loss is safe and reasonable.

For long-duration events, such as a century bike ride, the average rider will also lose a pound or more in energy stores (glycogen, fat, and muscle tissue) in addition to the water, so figure that into your weight difference.

ounces, that you should aim for daily. Metrically, you'll multiply your body weight in kilograms by about 33-39 and that'll give you a good estimate, in milliliters, of what you should be drinking daily. Caveat: If you have not been following this recommendation consistently, you'll want to start increasing your daily water consumption gradually until you reach your target amount. If you increase your fluid intake too quickly it will overwhelm your body with too much fluid too soon, which may increase the potential for hyponatremia.

For satisfying hydration requirements prior to a workout or race, there have been a number of recommendations presented over the years. These are the two that we believe to be the most sensible, the ones that will satisfy hydration needs without putting you at the risk for overhydration:

• One liter of fluid (about 34 ounces) in the two hours prior to the start (about 17 ounces/500 milliliters per hour), ceasing consumption about 20-30 minutes before you begin the workout or race.

• 10-12 ounces (approx 295-355 milliliters) of fluid each hour up to 30 minutes prior to the start (24-30 ounces total fluid intake). Keep in mind that even though these are our recommendations, you need to determine what works best for your system and the particular logistics of the race or training session ahead.

Personalized data is the key to hydration efficiency

If you've spent money on a heart rate monitor, a multi-function watch, or a body fat measuring device, and if you use them properly, you already have some serious training tools. We suggest that a good scale (preferably one that can measure less than one pound increments, such as a balance scale) may well prove to be your most valuable fitness investment. Weigh yourself before and after each outing, carefully noting the time, exertion level, miles, weather, and fluid, fuel, and electrolyte consumption. Another low-tech hint: make sure you know the capacity of your water bottles and hydration packs. Once you begin to log your fluid consumption and weight fluctuations, you'll have the data to accurately calculate your personal needs in this absolutely vital area.

We don't offer any "one size fits all" remedies. We do offer prudent and scientifically substantiated advice. Each athlete is personally responsible for including hydration, fueling, and electrolyte replacement in his or her training program. We have given you some guidelines to start your assessment and calculation of your personal hydration needs. You must find out in practice—before competition— what works for you. Most will find that your final figures will come very close to our suggested starting points. For others, you might find that in certain instances your needs for a particular event will require substantial modification.

SUMMARY

Dehydration and overhydration are common problems that plague far too many athletes, some with severe consequences. Armed with the guidelines contained in this article, along with practice and testing in training, your performance and health need not suffer. Instead, you'll be ahead of the vast majority of athletes who continue to make the same mistakes over and over again.

ELECTROLYTE REPLENISHMENT

Why it's so important and how to do it right

*Blake Bjornson hammers at the Whitefish Lake Triathlon.
Photo : Angela Miller*

Highly variable and highly important

1. **Electrolyte needs vary much more widely than fluids and calories**, among athletes in general, and also for the individual athlete training/racing under differing conditions.

2. **You will need to determine your usage for weather conditions, duration, and intensity of exercise.** Log your consumption and the variables of each training session. Soon you'll know what works best for you under various conditions.

3. Whatever your consumption, **you must use a supplement that includes a full panel of electrolytes**, not just salt (sodium) and potassium.

4. Make sure that your overall dietary intake of sodium is low.

Besides contributing to many health problems, **high-sodium diets encourage faster sodium depletion during exercise.**

5. **We recommend that as a start, you try 1-3 Endurolytes capsules/ scoops or 0.5-1.5 Endurolytes Fizz per hour**, and adjust from there.

6. **For light and/or short duration exercise, the modest electrolyte component in HEED might be sufficient.**

7. **NEVER, ever, use salt tablets.** Never.

Start reading the full article on page 40

INTRODUCTION

Electrolytes are analogous to the motor oil in your car—they don't make the engine run, but they're absolutely necessary to keep everything running smoothly. Proper functioning of the digestive, nervous, cardiac, and muscular systems depends on adequate electrolyte levels.

Muscle cramping, though there are many theories as to why it happens, usually involves improper hydration and/or improper electrolyte replenishment. No one wants to cramp, of course, but remember, cramping is a place far down the road of electrolyte depletion. Cramping is your body's painful way of saying "Hey! I'm on empty! Resupply me now or I'm going to stop!" It's like the oil light on the dash; you never want it to get that low.

That's precisely why, just as you shouldn't wait until you bonk before you refuel, or you're dehydrated before you replenish fluids, you shouldn't wait for cramps to remind you to take electrolytes.

In this article, we'll look closely at this vital, but often neglected and misunderstood, aspect of fueling. We'll tell you why salt tablets don't work and why Endurolytes is unquestionably the finest electrolyte formula available.

FULL ARTICLE

Proper fueling during exercise requires more than replenishing calories and fluids; it involves consistent and adequate electrolyte support as well. Electrolyte needs vary much more than either caloric or hydration needs, so you will have to experiment quite a bit in training until you have this aspect of your fueling tailored to your specific requirements under various conditions.

What are electrolytes? Why do I need them?

Electrolytes are chemicals that form electrically charged particles (ions) in body fluids. These ions carry the electrical energy necessary for many functions, including muscle contractions and transmission of nerve impulses. Many bodily functions depend on electrolytes; optimal performance requires a consistent and adequate supply of these important nutrients.

Many athletes neglect consistent electrolyte replenishment because they've "never had cramping problems." Even if you've been fortunate enough to have never suffered the painful, debilitating effects of cramping, you still need to provide your body with a consistent and adequate supply of electrolytes. Why? Because the goal in replenishing electrolytes is not so

What about salt tablets?

Salt tablets are an unacceptable choice for electrolyte replenishment for two reasons:

1. They provide only two of the electrolytes your body requires—sodium and chloride.

2. They can oversupply sodium, thereby overwhelming the body's complex mechanism for regulating sodium.

Read the indepth explanation in the full article below.

· ·

Article continues here

much to prevent cramping, but to maintain specific bodily functions at optimal levels. Cramping is your body's way of letting you know that, in terms of electrolytes, it's "on empty." When you've reached that point, your performance has been severely compromised for some time. Remember, you want your body to perform smoothly, without interruption or compromise, so just as you shouldn't wait until you're dehydrated or bonking before you replenish fluids or calories, you never want to wait until you're cramping before replenishing electrolytes. Consistent replenishment of electrolytes is just as important as the fuel you consume and the water you drink during exercise.

Can't I just use salt tablets?

Salt tablets are unacceptable for the two reasons listed above. Each of these issues are important, and we'll discuss both of them. Right now, let's focus primarily on the second one.

Far too many athletes have suffered needlessly with swollen hands and feet from water retention due to ingestion of salt tablets or electrolyte products too high in sodium during prolonged exercise in the heat. The body has very effective mechanisms to regulate and recirculate sodium from body stores. Excess sodium consumption interferes with or neutralizes these complex mechanisms. Sweat generates large sodium losses, which is monitored closely through hormonal receptors throughout the body. However, rapid sodium replacement neutralizes the system, allowing water intake to dilute the sodium content. High-sodium electrolyte supplementation contravenes

▶ The truth is that the human body needs only a minute amount of sodium to function normally.

▶ We require a mere 500 mg of sodium each day; athletes maybe 2,000 mg, which is easily supplied by natural, unprocessed foods.

▶ The average American consumes approximately 6,000-8,000 mg per day, well above the upper end recommended dose of 2,300-2,400 mg/day.

▶ The average athlete stores at least 8,000 mg of dietary sodium in tissues and has these stores available during exercise.

the natural physiological control of serum electrolytes, and once the body detects an increase in sodium from exogenous sources (i.e., food, salt tablets, or products too high in sodium), the hormone aldosterone signals the kidneys to stop filtering and recirculating sodium. Instead, the kidneys will excrete sodium; another hormone, vasopressin, will predominate and cause fluid retention. While ingesting large amounts of sodium may temporarily resolve a sodium deficiency, doing so substantially increases the risk of a number of problems, including increased fluid storage and thus swelling, or edema, in the distal extremities, elevated blood pressure, and increased rate of sodium excretion. All of these inhibit performance. If you've ever finished a workout or race with swollen hands, wrists, feet, or ankles, or if you have experienced puffiness under your eyes and around your cheeks, chances are your sodium/salt intake was too high.

The truth is that the human body needs only a minute amount of sodium to function normally. We require a mere 500 mg of sodium each day; athletes maybe 2,000 mg, which is easily supplied by natural, unprocessed foods. However, the average American consumes approximately 6,000-8,000 mg per day, well above the upper end recommended dose of 2,300-2,400 mg/day.* *(See asterik on page 44)* The average athlete stores at least 8,000 mg of dietary sodium in tissues and has these stores available during exercise. In other words, you already have a vast reservoir of sodium available in your body from your diet, ready to serve you during

Article continues on page 44

Sodium imbalance may lead to poor performance

What we found

We've repeatedly observed the following characteristics in endurance athletes who reported symptoms of severe sodium imbalance during or immediately following races or workouts:

1. Dietary sodium intake above 6,000 mg/day.

2. Fluid consumption in excess of 30 oz/hour (approx 890 ml/hr).

3. Food consumption in excess of 300 cal/hour.

4. Failure to acclimatize to hyperthermic (hot weather) conditions, including at least one workout of 60% or greater of the event distance.

What to do

You can diminish performance-inhibiting problems of excess sodium consumption by:

1. Reducing your dietary intake of sodium to 2,300 mg/day or lower. This not only aids performance, it's a substantially healthier dietary procedure.

2. Limit your fluid intake during exercise to 20-25 oz/hour (590-740 ml/hr).

3. Consume an appropriate amount of calories during exercise. For most athletes this is an intake of 240-280/hour, though it is oftentimes even less.

4. Train two to three weeks in the same heat or humidity as the event.

Bottom line

Salty foods and/or salt tablets will not cut it when it comes to electrolyte replenishment. Instead, adopt a low-sodium approach that emphasizes a balance of essential minerals that cooperatively enhance the body's natural hormone and enzyme actions. You want a product that will provide comprehensive electrolyte support without compromising internal regulation.

Article continues here

The Fast Lane

....

▶ Not only are high-sodium diets bad for your health, but those who consume high amounts of sodium in their diet are guaranteed greater sodium loss rates and require greater sodium intakes during exercise.

....

▶ The body is able to replace, at best, only about one-third of what it loses during exercise; this is true for fluids, calories, and electrolytes.

....

▶ If you try to replace in equal amounts all of the electrolytes you lose, a number of hormonal triggers may create all sorts of problems such as gastric distress, edema, muscle spasms, and cramping.

....

....

* Article Reference
"LESS IS BEST–The right way to fuel"
Page 12

....

exercise. In addition, your body has a highly complex and efficient way of monitoring and recirculating sodium back into the blood, which it does to maintain homeostasis. You do need to replenish sodium during exercise, but you must do so with amounts that cooperate with, and do not override, these complex body mechanisms.

In 2009, data from the U.S. Centers for Disease Control and Prevention provided additional scientific evidence that the majority of Americans over the age of twenty should limit the amount of sodium (salt) they consume daily to 1,500 milligrams (mg) to prevent and reduce high blood pressure.

High sodium health consequences

Not only are high-sodium diets bad for your health, but those who consume large amounts of sodium in their diet are guaranteed greater sodium loss rates and require greater sodium intakes during exercise. Sodium, as you probably know, drives thirst, and thirst drives drinking until excess results . . . definitely not a performance-enhancing scenario.

Don't I need to replace what I sweat out?

It's easy to formulate a product that matches one of the many perspiration analysis studies and then sell it on the basis that athletes simply need to replace what they lose. Some products do just that. Unfortunately, there's a problem with this because individual sweat-loss differences vary greatly, and the human body does not and cannot efficiently replace what it expends during exercise at any intensity above a walking pace. Electrolytes lost are not replaced by electrolytes consumed.

The body is able to replace, at best, only about one-third of what it loses during exercise; this is true for fluids, calories, and

Thoughts on reducing sodium

"Limiting sodium is recommended since research supports that chronic consumption of more than 2,300 milligrams per day may contribute to congestive heart failure (CHF), hypertension, muscle stiffness, edema, irritability, osteoarthritis, osteoporosis, pre-menstrual syndrome (PMS), liver disorders, ulcers, and cataracts."

- William Misner, Ph.D. - Director of Research & Product Development, Emeritus

Article continues here

electrolytes. If you try to replace all the fluids at once, you may end up with dilutional hyponatremia (overly diluted blood sodium levels) or water intoxication. If you attempt to replace all the fuel you expend, your stomach will back up in total rebellion, and refueling will grind to a halt. Likewise, if you try to replace in equal amounts all of the electrolytes you lose, a number of hormonal triggers may create all sorts of problems such as gastric distress, edema, muscle spasms, and cramping.

As emphasized in the "LESS IS BEST–The right way to fuel"* article at the beginning of this book, the key to successful fueling (fluids, calories, and electrolytes) is to NOT focus on what you lose, but rather on how much your body can effectively accept and absorb. Bill Misner, Ph.D., says, "Give it [your body] 30-40%, even though it cries aloud for 110%." When it comes to the amount of fluids you drink, calories you eat, and electrolytes

you replenish, this is an absolutely vital principle to remember. The closer you adhere to it, the greater your opportunity for success.

Pre-loading sodium prior to a race? Bad idea!

Courtesy of an article written by a registered dietician, one practice now being considered, and even adopted by many athletes, is to "... increase sodium in the diet by pre-loading three to four grams of sodium about 12 to 24 hours before the race."

What is bothersome about this recommendation is that one would think that a registered dietician ought to be well-versed on the health consequences of a high-sodium diet (which the overwhelming majority of Americans consume). Yet this particular person advocates additional sodium in the diet prior to a race. The question is: "Is this a

A number of references are provided in the article, apparently to solidify these recommendations:

1) Eichner, E.R. "Genetic and Other Determinants of Sweat Sodium." Current Sports Medicine Reports 7.4 Supp 1(2008): 236-S40.

Comment: Our interpretation of Eichner's statements/conclusions is that the more sodium in the pre-event diet, the more plasma aldosterone level is suppressed, resulting in a higher rate of sodium loss in sweat during the event. Our position is that suppression of aldosterone prior to events by increasing sodium intake is counterproductive to keeping natural body homeostatic controls in the healthy norm range, which means consuming a low sodium diet of under 2,300 mg daily.

Bottom line: More sodium in the diet equals more sodium lost during exercise.

2) Murray, R. and L. Kenney, "Sodium Balance and Exercise." Current Sports Medicine Reports 7.4 Supp. 1 (2008): S1-S2.

Comment: Our position is that over 2,300 mg/day results in harmful consequences to health proportionate to predisposed individual sensitivity, while a large majority of the human population reacts negatively to >5,800 mg/day.

Bottom line: Keeping sodium intake levels between 1,500-2,300 mg/day will support sodium requirements without taxing the aldosterone pathway or the kidney organ's role in homeostasis.

3) Stachenfeld, N.S. "Acute Effects of Sodium Ingestion on Thirst and Cardiovascular Function." Current Sports Medicine Reports 7.4 Supp. 1(2008): S7-S13.

The Fast Lane

▶ The body has a very complex and effective way of monitoring, recirculating, and thus conserving its stores of sodium.

▶ More sodium in the diet equals more sodium lost during exercise.

▶ Keeping sodium intake levels between 1,500-2,300 mg/day will support sodium requirements without taxing the aldosterone pathway or the kidney organ's role in homeostasis.

▶ A low-sodium diet and a more conservative sodium intake—in tandem with other depleting electrolytes—during a workout or race creates an environment where lower amounts of sodium are lost in sweat and urine.

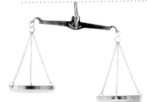

Sodium imbalance: what it causes and how to fix it, page 43

Comment: The human body is constructed to be sensitive in monitoring homeostatic electrolyte balance. This suggests that a consistent intake of small amounts of fluids and electrolytes help to prevent severe deficits of fluids and loss of electrolytes.

How the body controls serum sodium

Aldosterone is a hormone that controls the rate of sodium circulated in the human body. When sodium levels dip too low, via loss in perspiration or urine, aldosterone is released, stimulating the kidney tubule cells to increase re-absorption of sodium back into the blood. In basic terms, the body has a very complex and effective way of monitoring, recirculating, and thus conserving its stores of sodium.

High sodium intake will suppress serum aldosterone, whereas low sodium intake will elevate serum aldosterone. In other words, too much sodium—be it via diet and/or during exercise—will suppress and neutralize aldosterone's sodium recirculation (and thus sparing) effects, causing more sodium to be lost. Conversely, a low-sodium diet and a more conservative sodium intake—in tandem with other depleting electrolytes—during a workout or race creates an environment where lower amounts of sodium are lost in sweat and urine.

This is also why "sweat rate" figures can be deceiving. You'll find many a coach or researcher stating something to the effect of "I've seen athletes lose up to several grams of sodium during a one-hour training session." That may very well be true for some athletes during such a short-duration bout of exercise, especially if it's under a controlled environment (such as riding a stationary bike in a warm

Keep your electrolytes in check with Endurolytes. Photo : Kelly Pris

▶ Lowering your sodium intake in the diet—keeping it in the range of 2,300 mg or less—is not only a more appropriate recommendation/protocol for general health purposes, it will also benefit athletic performance as well.

▶ Remember, electrolyte intake needs to be below systemic detection, yet help alleviate systemic depression.

▶ Endurolytes is a full-spectrum electrolyte product designed to fulfill the body's electrolyte requirements. A good starting does is:

- Lighter weight athletes: 1-2 capsule or scoops/hour or 0.5-1 tablets/hour

- Medium weight athletes: 2-3 capsules or scoops/hour or 1-1.5 tablets/hour

- Larger athletes: 4-6 capsules or scoops/hour or 2-3 tablets/hour

room with no circulating air). However, that doesn't mean that those losses are sustainable hour after hour; again, the body's built-in chemical messengers and hormones (namely aldosterone) help prevent those losses from continuing down the same path. Yes, the body does need sodium replenishment but it has to be an amount that works in cooperation with aldosterone's "sodium recirculation/conservation" effects. A high-sodium diet and/or too-high sodium intake during a workout or race effectively negates aldosterone's desired effects, which means greater sodium losses.

Bottom line: Instead of adopting a recommendation that more and more sodium be added to the already too-high and unhealthy amounts in the diet, athletes should focus more on lowering their daily sodium intake. It is almost virtually guaranteed that each and every one of us consumes far more sodium than we need on a daily basis, and the harmful effects of oversupplying the body with sodium above its daily needs is a real and present danger which will compromise optimal health. Lowering your sodium intake in the diet—keeping it in the range of 2,300 mg or less—is not only a more appropriate recommendation/protocol for general health purposes, it will also benefit athletic performance as well. Definitely do not pre-load sodium in the days leading up to a race.

So what is the answer? How should I replenish electrolytes?

Proper electrolyte replenishment during endurance exercise requires a gradual, consistent approach that incorporates all of the electrolytes in amounts that do not override normal body mechanisms. Remember, electrolyte intake needs to be below systemic detection, yet help alleviate systemic depression. This means that you need to consume enough to support body functions and prevent heat-related

Where do I start?

Suggested amounts of Endurolytes (Capsules, Powder, and Fizz)

Electrolyte expenditure, and thus replenishment, varies tremendously between athletes, and it can also vary considerably for one athlete during the course of an event. Sweat composition studies performed by Shephard, Noakes, Costill, Moody, and others, have shown in a variety of stress exercise forms that an acclimatized, fit athlete loses half of the electrolytes and fluids as an un-acclimatized, unfit athlete does. Event-specific training in both duration and intensity halve electrolyte and fluid requirements in an endurance event. Body weight, fitness level, weather conditions, acclimatization level, and biological predisposition all greatly affect electrolyte depletion and the need for replenishment. That's why the hourly Endurolytes dose can range from 1-6 capsules, 1-6 scoops, or 0.5-3 tablets.

That being said, a good starting dose to consider is:

- **Lighter weight athletes:**
  1-2 capsules or scoops/hr or 0.5-1 tablets/hr
- **Medium weight athletes:**
  2-3 capsules or scoops/ hr or 1-1.5 tablets/hr
- **Larger athletes:**
  4-6 capsules or scoops/hr or 2-3 tablets/hr

Remember though, these are only suggested starting doses and the amount you need may be different, and may vary from hour to hour.

. . . .

Article continues here

issues such as cramping without overwhelming your body; electrolyte intake must slip under the body's "radar detection system" while still providing optimal support.

Endurolytes, Endurolytes Fizz, and Endurolytes Powder are full-spectrum electrolyte products designed to fulfill the body's electrolyte requirements, countering the effects of hyperthermia, optimizing specific bodily functions, and enhancing endurance performance, especially beyond the two-hour mark. The electrolyte profile of the Endurolytes

formula balances cations (positively charged ions) and anions (negatively charged ions) responsibly without emphasizing one electrolyte over others. This is a key note to remember: When a balance of electrolytes of cations to anions are managed in the energy producing cell—assuming the cell has adequate fuel and fluid—such a cell will produce energy at a higher rate than one overdosed by a single cation mixed with an irrational list of anions. That's a darn good reason to avoid going "salt only" or to use products—be they fuels or supplements—that

What about HEED?

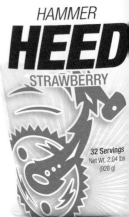

HEED is Hammer Nutrition's complex carbohydrate powdered sports drink. One of the nice features of HEED is that it contains a complete and easily assimilated electrolyte profile, not just salt and potassium, which is all you get in most other sports drinks. Each scoop of HEED provides the electrolyte equivalent of one Endurolytes capsule. Some athletes will find that with a scoop or two of HEED in their water bottle, they're good for an hour or more. For other athletes, the electrolyte profile in HEED will provide an excellent base from which additional Endurolytes capsules can be consumed (or Endurolytes Fizz or Endurolytes Powder can be added to the mix) to completely satisfy electrolyte needs.

The Fast Lane

▶ Each person has a unique biological predisposition in terms of minerals lost via perspiration.

▶ The differences in an athlete's size and fitness, as well as the pace of exercise, and of course the humidity and heat, can mean up to a 1,000% difference when one athlete's sweat rate is compared to another's.

▶ A "one-size-fits-all" formula based merely on sweat rates cannot, and will not, adequately support your specific electrolyte requirements.

Article continues here

contain high levels of sodium, especially at the expense of too-low amounts of other electrolytic minerals. Additionally, we do not formulate Endurolytes, Endurolytes Fizz, and Endurolytes Powder to reflect the amounts of electrolyte loss in sweat because each person has a unique biological predisposition in terms of minerals lost via perspiration. Furthermore, the differences in an athlete's size and fitness, as well as the pace of exercise, and of course the humidity and heat, can mean up to a 1000% difference when one athlete's sweat rate is compared to another's. A "one size fits all" formula based merely on sweat rates cannot, and will not, adequately support your specific electrolyte requirements.

In the purest sense, the Endurolytes formula is not so much an electrolyte replacement product, but is better described as an "electrolyte stress support formula." It helps the body perform better under the demands of exercise, especially in heat, by providing a full complement of minerals in the proper balance without interfering with normal body control systems.

SUMMARY

Consistent replenishment of fluids and calories is essential to maintain energy levels during workouts and races. Providing constant replenishment of electrolytes is an equally important component of proper fueling.

Getting your fluid and caloric needs dialed in and nailed down is fairly easy to accomplish, but fulfilling your electrolyte needs requires more attention because you have much more variability to account for. Using Endurolytes, Endurolytes Fizz, or Endurolytes Powder in your training will resolve that challenge. They contain the right minerals in the right balance, and because they are independent of your caloric and hydration sources, they provide you with the necessary dosing flexibility. Regardless of your size, sport, training intensity, fitness level, or the weather, you can fulfill your electrolytic mineral needs accurately and precisely hour after hour with Endurolytes, Endurolytes Fizz, or Endurolytes Powder.

The Hammer Nutrition website has several detailed articles on sodium and electrolyte replenishment. We especially recommend:

"The Endurolytes Rationale" (www.hammernutrition.com/za/ HNT?PAGE=ARTICLE&ARTICLE. ID=770)

"Does a High Sodium Diet Inhibit Endurance Performance and Health?" (www.hammernutrition.com/za/ HNT?PAGE=ARTICLE&ARTICLE. ID=4892)

"What is the Role of Sodium During Hyperthermic Endurance Events?" (www.hammernutrition.com/ downloads/JOE/nov05.pdf)

The Endurolytes formula

Endurolytes contains chelated minerals. Chelation is the process of bonding a mineral to another substance, ideally an amino acid, making the mineral more bioavailable. Chelated minerals are the form most often recommended because they provide greater absorption than their non-chelated counterparts. For example, magnesium is 87% absorbed when chelated, but only 16% when taken in an inorganic, non-chelated form. One nutritional scientist wrote, "Estimates of normal mineral absorption average 10%; however, absorption of chelated minerals may be as high as 60%." Let's examine each mineral . . .

CALCIUM is the most abundant mineral in the human body (about 2.85 lbs/.8 kg in the average person). Normal heart rhythm, healthy nerve transmission, and strong muscle contractions require a constant blood calcium level. During exercise, calcium-dependent enzymes produce energy from fatty and amino acid conversion. Because fatty acids are such an important fuel during endurance exercise, providing 60-65% of your energy needs when exercise goes beyond two hours in length, having adequate calcium available to efficiently convert them into energy is crucial. When blood calcium runs low, the body extracts it from the bones, but this process can't keep up with your exercise depletion rate. Serum calcium deficiency during endurance events may produce high blood pressure, muscle cramps, and weakness.

MAGNESIUM should accompany calcium at a ratio of 1:2. When calcium flows into working muscle cells, the muscle contracts; when calcium leaves and magnesium replaces it, the muscle relaxes. Many enzymatic reactions necessary for fuel conversion to muscular energy occur in the presence of adequate magnesium. Deficiency of magnesium contributes to muscle cramps, tremors, sleep disturbances, and in some cases, convulsive disorders.

POTASSIUM is the chief cation (positively charged ion) within all muscle cells. It is necessary for maintaining the optimal concentration and balance of sodium. Potassium deficiency symptoms are nausea, vomiting, muscle weakness, muscle spasms, cramping, and rapid heart rate. Even though 100-200 mg are lost in sweat alone (not counting internal muscle and cell use), if we try to replace those amounts all at once, optimal sodium balance is altered. In addition, too much potassium is hard on the stomach and can cause severe stomach distress.

SODIUM is the chief cation (positively charged ion) outside the cell. The average

American carries 8,000 mg of excess sodium in extracellular tissues. During endurance events, a minimum of three to four hours is necessary to deplete this mineral, which may result in symptoms of abnormal heartbeat, muscle twitching, and hypoventilation. However, if sodium is replaced at or near the same rate as depletion, it overrides the hormonal regulating mechanisms that enable the body to conserve electrolytes. Consumption of too much sodium will cause a variety of problems, the least of which is fluid retention. Therefore, we highly recommend a more moderate, body-cooperative replenishment of sodium.

CHLORIDE is the relative anion (negatively charged ion) that accompanies sodium. This electrolyte is absolutely necessary in maintaining the osmotic tension in both blood and extracellular fluids. It's a somewhat complicated process, but to put it in the simplest terms, think of osmotic tension as being the proper balance and consistency of body fluids and electrolytes. An appropriate amount of chloride (as sodium chloride) supports, but does not override, the function of the hormone aldosterone in regulating and conserving proper electrolyte levels.

MANGANESE is included in Endurolytes as it is necessary in trace amounts for optimal muscle cell enzyme reactions for conversion of fatty acids and protein into energy. Again, fatty acids and protein are a crucial part of the endurance athlete's fuel supply, so while manganese is not technically an electrolyte, its importance cannot be overstated. Research also shows that manganese deficiency plays a key role in blood sugar fluctuation, free radical build-up from intense exercise, and nerve function disorders, especially in older athletes.

PYRIDOXINE HCL (vitamin B-6) is a coenzyme required in 60 enzymatic reactions involving metabolism of carbohydrates, fats, and protein. We include this water-soluble B vitamin in Endurolytes because of its active role in maintaining sodium-potassium balance.

L-TYROSINE is an amino acid added to the Endurolytes formula to protect thyroid and adrenal function. Blood plasma deficiency during extreme endurance events will lower thyroid and adrenal production, which hinders the proper rate of metabolism. Symptoms of I-tyrosine depletion first appear as depression, later anger, then despondency that degenerates into total despair. If any of these has ever happened to you during a long training session or race, it may be due to low thyroid and adrenal production; it can be easily avoided by the intake of supplemental I-tyrosine via any of the Endurolytes products.

GLYCINE is an amino acid added to Endurolytes Powder to help neutralize the naturally salty/bitter taste of the minerals.

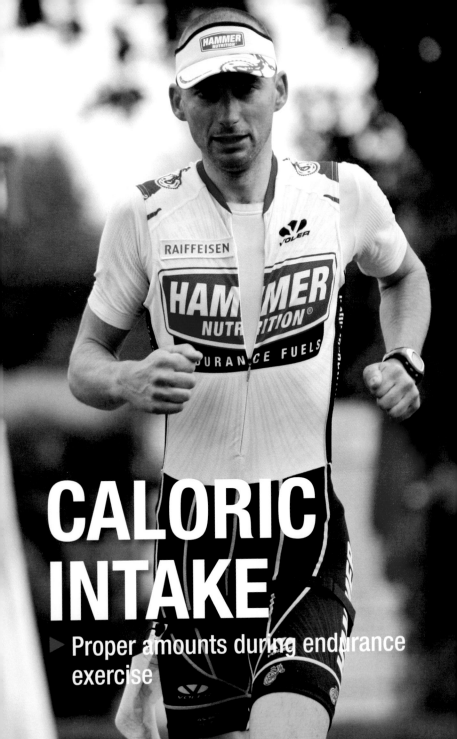

CALORIC INTAKE

▶ Proper amounts during endurance exercise

Calories count!

1. **During endurance exercise, you will expend on the order of 600-900 cal/hr. Does this mean that you should consume that much to keep your energy level up? Absolutely not**, because your body cannot absorb and process calories at that rate.

2. **The limiting factors in caloric replenishment are gastric emptying and liver metabolism of carbohydrates. For most athletes, this is in the 240-280 cal/hr range, and this, by and large, sets the limit of caloric intake.** If you consume more than that, you will most likely exerience some form of stomach distress.

3. **Is this several hundred cal/hr energy deficit a big problem? No, because your body converts stored fat to energy to make up the shortfall.** Plus, if you are a serious athlete who has properly managed your training, fueling, and recovery, you will have a full supply of muscle glycogen, your body's "premium" fuel, when you start.

4. **Fueling and supplementation strategies can increase your fats-to-fuels conversion capability.**

5. **For races and training up to two hours in duration—perhaps stretched out as far as three hours —you can rely on carbohydrates alone (Hammer Gel or HEED) for your fuel; anything longer and you will need to add some protein to your fuel** or your body will begin to cannibalize its own muscle tissue for energy. Soy is the protein of choice for this application.

6. **Hammer Nutrition's Sustained Energy and Perpetuem are the premiere long-distance fuels as** they contain both complex carbs and soy protein.

7. **Avoid any drink or mix that uses simple sugars as an energy source. Your body cannot absorb adequate calories in the form of simple sugars.** Also, simple sugars are a poor fuel source as they cause energy spikes and crashes. Use complex carbs only for your fuels.

Start reading the full article on page 56

INTRODUCTION

In this article you'll learn the right way to deal with the three critical elements of endurance fueling: what kind of fuel to consume, how much, and when. The answers may surprise you, but I can promise that if you adopt and apply these fueling guidelines, you will see noticeably positive results. You put great effort into your training and spend a significant amount of money acquiring the best equipment, so make sure your fueling strategy is equally top of the line. Your body will thank you and your performance will be the proof.

FULL ARTICLE

Endurance and ultra-endurance athletes require all three forms of fuel that the human body uses for energy: carbohydrate, protein, and fat. A major factor for optimal performance is using the right fuel, at the right time, in the right amount. Like every aspect of success in endurance events, proper nutrition requires planning, practice, and training to reap the benefits on race day. This article will give you the background information you need about fueling.

As all athletes know, "carbs are king" when it comes to fueling the body for any endurance exercise. That does not mean, however, that any carbohydrate at any time will keep you going. Carbohydrates can either help or hinder performance, depending on what kind you use, how much you use, and when you use them. Far too many misinformed athletes continue to use energy products loaded with simple sugars, or they use complex carbs, a superior choice, but at the wrong time and in the wrong amounts. These practices will actually impair, not help, your performance.

Simple sugars, maltodextrin, and osmolality

Most dietary sugars are simple molecules known as monosaccharides and disaccharides. The shorter the chain length of a carbohydrate source, the higher it will raise a chemical measure known as osmolality when dissolved. In solution, simple sugars can only attain about 6-8% concentration or they will sit undigested in your stomach, as the osmolality will be incompatible with the digestive juices. Products containing simple sugars, typically sucrose, fructose, and/or glucose (dextrose), must be extremely diluted to match body fluid osmolality (280-303 mOsm). This weak of a concentration presents a problem to athletes because it cannot provide sufficient calories (perhaps only 100 cal/hour, at the most) to working muscles. To obtain enough calories from a weak 6-8% solution, an athlete would have to consume two or more bottles of fuel per hour, which means excess fluids, increasing the risk of fluid intoxication. Using simple sugar-based "energy drinks" is not a wise strategy.

"Well then," you might say, "I'll just mix a stronger concentration." But this approach also fails. Making a double or triple strength mixture from a simple sugar-based carbohydrate fuel won't work because the concentration of that mixture will exceed 6-8%, far too concentrated to match body fluid osmolality. It will remain in the stomach until sufficiently diluted, which may cause substantial stomach distress. Drinking more water to dilute your over-concentrated concoction puts you back in the original condition of increased risk of overhydration and all the problems that causes, so it's not a good option. But if you don't drink more, your body

The fact is that using simple sugar-based products—either by themselves or in tandem with complex carbohydrate products—is futile! Endurance athletes who try to fulfill calorie/energy requirements with sugar-based drinks, gels, and powder mixes usually end up with a variety of complaints and poor performances.

The Hammer Bar that Scott carried to 22,841' hit the spot on the summit of Aconcagua in Chile.
Photo : courtesy of Scott Holder

The Fast Lane

▶ Based on caloric delivery alone, complex carbohydrates such as maltodextrin are far superior to simple carbohydrates (simple sugars).

▶ Maltodextrin allows you to absorb a greater volume of calories for use as energy than you can from simple sugars.

▶ We include only complex carbohydrates in Hammer Nutrition fuels. They contain no added simple sugars.

will draw fluids and electrolytes from other areas that critically need them (like blood and muscle) and divert them to the digestive system to lower the osmolality of your over-concentrated simple sugar drink. This will also result in a variety of stomach distresses, not to mention increased cramping potential and other performance-trashing issues.

The same problem occurs when an athlete combines a simple sugar fuel with a complex carbohydrate fuel. Consumed together or within close proximity of each other, simple sugars and complex carbohydrates increase the solution concentration beyond the efficient digestion level for either component. This will compromise energy production and promote the likelihood of a variety of stomach issues. In the words of Dr. Bill Misner, "Adding simple sugar fractions (any of the carbohydrates ending in "ose") to complex carbohydrate fractions (maltodextrins) may double the osmolar pressure of the solution to hypertonic values. When a 6-8% simple sugar solution is added to a 15-18% complex carbohydrate solution, the osmolality of the combined solutions is simply not absorbable in the human gut." Molecules that contain many sugar units chained together are called polysaccharides, known familiarly as complex carbs and starches. One of these, maltodextrin, can make up to an 18% solution concentration and still match digestive system osmolality. This allows very efficient passage from the digestive tract to the liver, which converts some of the maltodextrin to glycogen for storage and some directly to glucose for immediate use by the muscles. With polysaccharides you get much more energy from stomach to liver, thus providing maximal amounts of energy to be produced in a form that your body can efficiently process.

Based on caloric delivery alone, complex carbohydrates such as maltodextrin are far superior to simple carbohydrates (simple

Simple sugars = ineffective fuel

Read the label before you buy. If there's anything that ends in "ose" in the ingredient list, put it back!

Using simple sugars to fuel your body is like trying to heat your house by burning newspapers in your stove. You get a fast heat, but it burns out quickly, and you have to continually feed the fire. Not good! Complex carbohydrates, on the other hand, are similar to putting a nice big log on the fire in that they burn longer and more evenly, with the declination in "heat" (energy levels) being much more gradual.

The maltodextrins in Hammer Gel, HEED, Sustained Energy, Perpetuem, Perpetuem Solids, and Recoverite allow you to obtain the maximum amount of calories you need. They provide a more consistent and longer lasting energy supply without putting you at risk for stomach distress.

Article continues here

sugars). But that's not all. Simple sugars, even in small amounts, can incite a condition known as "insulin spike." This sudden recruitment of insulin causes a subsequent dramatic drop in blood sugar, which can take blood sugar levels even below the fasting level! This "flash and crash" type of energy typically results in the dreaded "bonk," something every athlete wants to avoid. However, complex carbs, which enter the bloodstream at a 15-18% solution, do not promote this wild fluctuation in blood sugar levels. Even though a maltodextrin might have a high GI (see next page) and rapidly elevate blood sugar levels (a desirable effect), during exercise your body processes them with far less insulin fluctuation, most likely due to the steady release and breakdown of glucose from its polymeric source, and other hormonal factors. You never get the below-baseline drop in blood glucose that simple sugars cause.

Some athletic nutritionists disregard osmolality, but we do not believe its importance

The Fast Lane

▶ Glycemic Index (GI) rates the speed at which the body breaks down a carbohydrate into glucose.

▶ The lower the GI, the slower the process, and therefore the more stable the energy release.

▶ For food eaten at times other than during exercise and recovery, we recommend eating foods with a low-to-middle GI rating.

▶ During and immediately following exercise, a high-GI carbohydrate—one that elevates blood sugar levels rapidly—is desirable.

▶ Maltodextrins raise blood insulin more effectively than simple sugars, but without the rapid and precipitous drop that is common with simple sugars.

can be overstated. As Dr. Misner states, "when osmolality goes above 303 or below 280 mOsm, the gut must pull minerals and fluids . . . to mediate a narrow 280-303 mOsm range for immediate calorie absorption." Both simple sugars and complex carbohydrate maltodextrins are absorbed at equal rates if the solution concentration matches body fluid osmolality (280-303 mOsm). Simple sugars meet this criterion only when they are mixed in calorically weak 6-8% concentrations; digestion slows down or ceases at higher concentrations. When athletes make a double or triple strength simple sugar-based drink, trying to increase caloric input, they usually develop problems such as gastric distress, bloating, flatulence, vomiting, and muscle cramps.

On the other hand, the maltodextrins (complex carbohydrates) used in Hammer Nutrition fuels match body fluid osmolality even when mixed in concentrations as high as 15-18%. This presents a distinct advantage because your body is able to digest, and thus convert to energy, a greater volume of calories from complex carbohydrates than it can from simple sugars.

Glycemic Index

People often ask about the glycemic index (GI) of various carbohydrates and how those figures relate to fueling for endurance exercise. Here's the scoop: GI rates the speed at which the body breaks down a carbohydrate into glucose. The lower the GI, the slower the process, and therefore the more stable the energy release. For food eaten at times other than during exercise and recovery, GI is an important dietary factor and we recommend eating foods with a low-to-middle GI rating.

However, during and immediately following exercise, a high-GI carbohydrate—one that elevates blood sugar levels rapidly—is desirable, as long as you keep caloric intake within approximately 280 cal/hour, as hormones associated with sympathetic nervous system activity will inhibit GI impact on insulin release. Negative diet/health-specific effects associated with consumption of high-GI carbohydrates are not a concern during and immediately after exercise; high-GI carbs actually perform better than low-GI carbs at these times.

Long-chain, high-GI maltodextrins have a GI value of about 130, compared to glucose (100) or sucrose (62). This means that maltodextrins raise blood insulin more effectively than simple sugars, but without the rapid and precipitous drop that is a common (and deleterious) effect of simple sugars. Also, as mentioned earlier, maltodextrins allow you to absorb a greater volume of calories than you can from simple sugars.

Don't complex carbs take longer to utilize?

Some suggest that since maltodextrin is many chains of glucose "hooked" together, it takes the body longer to break those chains down for conversion to glucose. In fact, one well-known triathlete contends that "your body uses sugar first before anything else so it makes sense to consume sugars like glucose."

Technically, this is true; all carbohydrates will eventually be broken down to glucose. However, the first fuel (sugar) the body will use when exercise commences is muscle-stored glycogen, which is a long-chain (complex) carbohydrate that, as Dr. Misner puts it: " . . . is a form of starch which contains eight parts amylopectin to two parts a-amylose." Thus, wouldn't it make

Mike Freeman, center, leads the group on an easy spin in Tucson.
Photo : Madeline Frank

The Fast Lane

▶ For better results, stick with complex carbohydrate fuels. Don't consume simple sugars with or within close proximity of complex carbohydrates.

▶ We do not recommend the use of multiple carbohydrate sources during exercise.

▶ After two decades of experience, we have found that in the overwhelming majority of the athletes we've worked with, the combination of simple sugars and long chain carbohydrates, and in amounts higher than approximately 1.0-1.1 grams per minute (roughly 4.0-4.6 calories per minute), have not yielded positive results. They did, however, increase performance-inhibiting, stomach-related maladies.

sense to say that if the body's first-used fuel is muscle glycogen and that its makeup is "complex" in nature, the body obviously is very efficient in breaking it down for rapid conversion to energy?

This particular athlete goes on to say, "As the race progresses, your ability to cleave it [maltodextrin] into the absorbable form of carbohydrate (glucose) gets slower and slower. But maltodextrin is patient. It will sit in your stomach and wait for quite a while for something to come along and break it into glucose. This, my friend, is what causes that very undesirable bloating and eventual feeling like you want to hurl."

We could not disagree more. Our unflinching belief is that the time it takes "from gut to muscle" isn't nearly as long as some "experts" think it is, if there is any difference to begin with. And even if maltodextrin took slightly longer in "breaking down in the gut" as compared to glucose—and the difference, if any, would be fractional— the earlier-mentioned benefits of using complex carbohydrates only versus simple sugars (such as glucose) or combinations of carbohydrates (which we'll discuss shortly) more than justifies the use of complex carbohydrates.

Interestingly, the very company this athlete is affiliated with (at least to some degree) states the following on their website: "Maltodextrin has a much lower osmolality than glucose and fructose and therefore can be mixed in much higher concentrations without any stomach issues. Molecules of maltodextrin are larger than glucose, so drinks with maltodextrin will have a few large particles compared to a drink with glucose. The number of particles determines how much water it will hold. The more molecules of smaller-sized glucose in the drink, the more water will be pulled into the intestine than the maltodextrin-based drink. Since maltodextrin-based products

Thoughts on caloric intake

"Absorption rate and how fast the liver can 'kick it out' are limiting factors. No matter what you eat, how much or how little, the body provides glucose to the bloodstream at a rate of about one gram/minute. Putting more calories in than can generate energy taxes gastric venues, electrolyte stores, and fluid levels."

- William Misner, Ph.D. - Director of Research & Product Development, Emeritus

Article continues here

don't pull as much water into the intestine, it is absorbed faster into the bloodstream."

Bottom line: While the process is, of course, quite detailed, the truth is that the bonds that compose maltodextrin are very weak and readily broken apart in the stomach. As already mentioned a couple of times now (but worth repeating again), maltodextrin allows you to absorb a greater volume of calories for use as energy than you can from simple sugars.

Complex carbohydrates only or a combination

of carbohydrate sources: Which is better for the endurance athlete?

Findings from research conducted by the Dutch sport scientist Asker Jeukendrup has caused quite a stir. In fact, a few companies produce fuels that contain the carbohydrate formulations used in the studies. In general, Jeukendrup found that a blend of

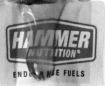

Rapid Energy Fuel

HAMMER NUTRITION® ENDURANCE FUELS

HAMMER GEL

RASPBERRY

▶ We have an enormous supply of calories in body fat. The typical athlete can count on a reserve of up to 100,000 calories in the form of stored fatty acids!

▶ Replenish calories in amounts that support efficient energy production and do not interfere with the use of fatty acids for fuel.

▶ After approximately 90-120 minutes, and continuing until you stop your activity, about 5-15% of your caloric utilization comes from protein.

carbohydrates increased oxidation rates, indicating higher energy production. In one study, cyclists who ingested a 2:1 mixture of maltodextrin to fructose oxidized carbohydrate up to 1.5 grams/minute. Another study used a mixture of glucose, fructose, and sucrose and had rates that peaked at 1.7 g/min. Both those results are pretty eye opening, considering that complex carbohydrates typically oxidize at a rate of about 1.0 g/min.

However, there's more to the results than what first meets the eye. Most of Jeukendrup's subjects cycled at low intensity, only 50-55% maximum power output, which I think we'd all agree is very much a recovery pace, if that.

To be blunt, at a leisurely 50% VO2 Max pace, athletes can digest cheeseburgers and pizza with no gastric issues. However, if the heart rate and core temperature are raised to only 70% VO2 Max, the body must divert core accumulated heat from central to peripheral. This reduces the blood volume available to absorb ingested carbohydrates or whatever the athlete has consumed. After over two decades of experience, we have found that in the overwhelming majority of the athletes we've worked with—athletes engaged in typical 75-85% efforts and/ or in multi-hour endurance events—the combination of simple sugars and long chain carbohydrates, and in amounts higher than approximately 1.0-1.1 grams per minute (roughly 4.0-4.6 calories per minute), have not yielded positive results. They did, however, increase performance-inhibiting, stomach-related maladies.

Lowell Greib, MSc ND, explains that gastric emptying is a key limiting step in carbohydrate metabolism: "If your stomach can't empty the product (no matter what it is) you are going to get nothing from it except a huge gut ache and possibly lots of vomiting! Unless there is new research that

THE BIG QUESTION : What should I consume?

In general, we recommend a range of **240-280 cal/hr.** Here's why . . .

You may be burning up to 800 cal/hr., but your body cannot replace that amount during exercise. Trying to replenish calories at the same rate as depletion only causes problems. Instead of having more energy available, you'll have a bloated stomach and perhaps even nausea and vomiting.

With some allowances provided for very large athletes, the average size* human body can only return, from the liver to muscle tissue, about 4.0-4.6 calories per minute, or about 240-280 cal/hr. Lighter weight athletes will need even less.

Most of the time, when you consume more than 280 cal/hr. during an event, the excess remains undigested in the stomach or passes unused into the bowel.

Approximately 160-165 lbs/72.5-75 kg

Article continues here

I am unaware of, gastric emptying is directly proportional to the osmolality of the solution in the stomach. Long chain carbohydrate (maltodextrin) contributes less to increasing the osmolality than do disaccharides (sucrose, lactose, maltose, etc.)."

The question is not whether or not Jeukendrup's published studies are disputable, but rather if these studies apply to faster paced, longer duration bouts of exercise. We do not believe this to be the case, which is why we do not recommend the use of multiple carbohydrate sources during exercise.

Bottom line: Stick with complex carbohydrate fuels, don't consume simple sugars with or within close proximity of complex carbohydrates, and we guarantee you'll see better results.

Fatty acids for fuel

If we can't replace all of the calories we expend, then how do we keep going hour after hour? The answer is that we have an enormous supply of calories in body fat. The typical athlete can count on a reserve of up to 100,000 calories in the form of stored fatty acids—that's enough,

The Fast Lane

▶ For exercise and competition that extends two hours or more, your primary fuel should incorporate protein in a ratio of about 8:1 (by weight) carbs to protein.

▶ The preferred protein for use during prolonged exercise is soy, primarily because its metabolization does not readily produce ammonia. Whey protein, with its high glutamine content, makes an excellent post-workout protein, but is not a good choice before or during exercise.

if you could process it all, to fuel a run from Portland, OR to Los Angeles, CA—a distance of almost 1,000 miles! These fatty acids are the fuel of choice when exercise goes beyond about two hours, providing approximately 60-65% of your caloric expenditure. In other words, your body has a vast reservoir of calories available from body fat stores and it will use those liberally to satisfy energy requirements during lengthy workouts and races.

However, for this process to continue without compromise or interruption, you must not consume excess calories. If you try to match energy losses with caloric replacement from your fuel, you will not only cause a variety of stomach-related ailments, you will also inhibit the efficient utilization of fats for fuel. The bottom line is that caloric donation from consumed fuels must cooperate with your internal fat-to-fuel conversion system. Do not attempt to completely replace caloric expenditure. Your best strategy is to replenish calories in amounts that support efficient energy production and do not interfere with the use of fatty acids for fuel.

Protein for fuel

Aside from certain circumstances, which we'll discuss shortly, when exercise goes beyond two hours, you need to incorporate some protein into the fuel mix. After approximately 90-120 minutes, and continuing until you stop your activity, about 5-15% of your caloric utilization comes from protein. This process, called gluconeogenesis, is unavoidable, and if you don't supply the needed protein in your fuel, your body will literally scavenge it from your own muscle tissue. This is called catabolism (muscle breakdown), known informally, but quite accurately, as "protein cannibalization." It can cause premature muscle fatigue (due to excess ammonia production from the protein breakdown process) as well as muscle depletion and post-exercise soreness. Protein cannibalization also compromises your immune system, leading to increased risk for colds, flu, and other diseases.

For exercise and competition that extends two hours or more, your primary fuel should incorporate protein in a ratio of about 8:1 (by weight) carbs to protein. Sustained Energy, Perpetuem, and Perpetuem Solids meet this requirement; they

- -

After approximately 90-120 minutes, and continuing until you stop your activity, about 5-15% of your caloric utilization comes from protein. This process, called gluconeogenesis, is unavoidable, and if you don't supply the needed protein in your fuel, your body will literally scavenge it from your own muscle tissue.

- -

are your best choices for fueling during any long-duration exercise.

The benefits of soy protein during endurance exercise

As noted previously, it's good to have a little protein along with your complex carbs to avoid the negative effects of muscle catabolism, but you must have the right kind of protein. The preferred protein for use during

prolonged exercise is soy, primarily because its metabolization does not readily produce ammonia. Whey protein, with its usually added amounts of glutamine, makes an excellent post-workout protein, but is not a good choice before or during exercise. You're already producing ammonia during exercise, so consuming glutamine supplements or glutamine-enhanced whey protein will only exacerbate the problem.

There is some confusion regarding the glutamine and ammonia build-up. Yes, glutamine does eventually scavenge ammonia. The key word, however, is "eventually." When glutamine metabolizes, it increases ammonia initially, then scavenges more than originally induced, but it takes approximately three hours or so to accomplish this. You're already producing ammonia during endurance exercise, and since ammonia is a primary culprit in premature fatigue, it seems logical that you'd not want to increase ammonia levels even more. However, that's exactly what you'll do when you consume glutamine supplements or glutamine-enhanced whey protein during exercise. That's one reason why soy protein is preferable for use during prolonged exercise.

Soy protein has a couple of other great features, too. First, it is an easily digestible protein. Second, it has an excellent amino acid profile, with a substantial proportion of branched chain amino acids, or

The Fast Lane

▶ A race that's in the 2-3 hour range, perhaps just slightly longer, is in a "gray area" so to speak, which means that you can use either a "carb + protein" fuel or a "carb only" fuel.

▶ Selection of fuel for a 2-3 hour training session or race, either carb only or carb + protein, should be based on the following:

- The type of race that you're doing

- The intensity of the effort

- The weather and how well you're acclimated to it

- The terrain

* Article Reference
"THE TOP 10–The
biggest mistakes
endurance athletes make"
Page 106

BCAAs, which your body readily converts for energy. During exercise, nitrogen is removed from BCAAs and used in the production of another amino acid, alanine, high amounts of which also occur naturally in soy protein. The liver converts alanine into glucose, which the bloodstream transports to the muscles for energy.

BCAAs and glutamic acid, another amino acid found in significant quantities in soy protein, also aid in the replenishing of glutamine within the body without the risk of ammonia production caused by orally ingested glutamine.

Soy's amino acid profile has high amounts of both alanine and histidine, which are the amino acid components of the dipeptide known as carnosine, a nutrient known for its antioxidant and acid buffering benefits. Soy protein also has a high level of aspartic acid, which plays an important role in energy production via the Krebs cycle. Additionally, soy protein has high levels of phenylalanine and tyrosine, both of which may aid in maintaining alertness during extreme ultra distance races.

Lastly, soy produces more uric acid than whey protein. This might not sound good, but uric acid is actually an antioxidant that helps neutralize the excessive free radicals produced during exercise. High uric acid levels, from soy's naturally occurring isoflavones, are another strong reason for preferring soy protein during endurance exercise.

The "gray area" of fueling

As discussed earlier, when exercise goes beyond two hours, we generally recommend that athletes use a "carb + protein" fuel (Sustained Energy or Perpetuem), either as their sole fuel from beginning to end, or as their primary fuel (roughly 2/3-3/4 of the time). The reason for this recommendation is that once you hit that second hour and beyond, a small percentage (roughly 5-15%) of energy requirements will be fulfilled from protein. If you don't provide some in the fuel mix, at least part of the time, your body has to cannibalize the lean muscle tissue to obtain the amino acids it needs to fulfill that small percentage of its energy requirements.

The last thing you want to do is have your body literally digest its own muscle tissue to make fuel. One reason is the increase in fatigue-causing ammonia; there is no doubt that excess ammonia is a primary culprit—perhaps THE primary culprit—in premature fatigue during endurance events. The other reason is that you'll have broken down a greater volume of muscle tissue, which will prolong recovery time.

Things may (key word "may") be a little different come race day. We believe that a race that's in the 2-3 hour range, perhaps just slightly longer, is in a "gray area" so to speak, which means that you can use either a "carb + protein" fuel (Sustained Energy or Perpetuem) or a "carb only" fuel (HEED or Hammer Gel). The selection needs to be based on the following:

• **The type of race that you're doing.** For example, running is a more impactive and thus a more "digestively challenging" type of exercise than cycling.

• **The intensity of the effort.** It's a lot easier to digest calories when the pace is more relaxed, which it usually is during a training session rather than during a race. That's why, in "THE TOP 10–The biggest mistakes endurance athletes make"* article, we suggest having a fueling game plan but to "write it in pencil, not in ink." What is meant by that saying is that caloric intakes that worked during training may not be appropriate during a race; you may need to consume slightly less in a race than you did during training. Increased anxiety, increased pace, and increased potential for dehydration all contribute to the possibility of a less-than-optimally-functioning

The Fast Lane

▶ Running is a more "digestively challenging" type of exercise than cycling.

It's a lot easier to digest calories when the pace is more relaxed.

The hotter the weather, the more compromised the digestive system becomes.

Doing lots of climbing usually diminishes digestive capabilities.

▶ If the race is going to be high intensity from the start and/ or the weather is going to be very warm-to-hot, a quick-to-digest fuel like Hammer Gel or HEED may be your best choice.

▶ Endurance Amino supplies your body with the primary amino acids that are used in the energy cycle.

digestive system. In addition, at the increased pace during a race, more blood is diverted from digestion and directed toward maintaining muscle performance.

• The weather and how well or poorly you're acclimated to it. The hotter the weather, the more compromised the digestive system becomes. During hot-weather racing, athletes usually find that they need to increase their water and Endurolytes intake while lowering their calorie intake.

• The terrain. For example, doing lots of climbing while on the bike or during a run usually diminishes digestive capabilities somewhat.

Our belief is that if the race is going to involve high intensity right from the gun, and/or if the weather is going to be very warm-to-hot, and/or if other factors such as hilly-to-mountainous terrain come into play, deference should be given to the fuel that is the quickest to digest, and that means HEED or Hammer Gel. Yes, some ammonia will be produced during the effort by not providing the body with some protein along with the carbs. However, if the race is in the 2-3 hour range—and perhaps just slightly longer—it will be over long before the issues involved with ammonia accumulation truly become problematic.

To summarize, we recommend a "carb + protein" drink (Sustained Energy or Perpetuem) when exercise goes beyond two or so hours. However, come race day—when a lot of variables need to be taken into consideration—you have a lot of options to choose from when the race is in the 2-3 hour range . . . you need to go with the fuel that makes the most sense, based on the aforementioned factors/variables. If those factors do come into play, we recommend the use of Hammer Gel or HEED for a high intensity race that's in the 2-3 hour range. If you know you're going to be out there for more than three hours we believe your body is going to perform better if Sustained Energy or Perpetuem is used as the primary-to-sole fuel, with the occasional use of Perpetuem Solids being perfectly acceptable as well.

All this said, this is not meant to be a "set in stone" rule. Everyone is different so your fuel selection may be different than another athlete's. The earlier-listed information is just a suggestion for you to consider when doing a race that is 2-3 hours in length—the "gray area" of fueling.

Endurance Amino - Where does it fit?

For these "gray area"-duration events, a HEED or Hammer Gel (or both), Endurolytes, and Endurance Amino combination is superb. You're supplying your body with high quality calories from two very easily digested fuel sources, you're taking care of electrolyte replenishment in ideal fashion via Endurolytes, and, with Endurance Amino, you're supplying your body with the primary amino acids (the three branched chain amino acids and alanine) that are used in the energy cycle. Plus, the BCAAs

in Endurance Amino assist in replenishing depleted glutamine stores while also helping to prevent muscle tissue breakdown, the latter helping to prevent excess fatigue-causing ammonia from being produced and accumulating. In addition, the glutathione component in Endurance Amino provides a number of benefits, primarily powerful antioxidant support.

During a "gray area"-duration event, you could certainly use Sustained Energy, Perpetuem, and Perpetuem Solids but for events in that 2-3 hour range it may be more feasible to use Hammer Gel or HEED to cover your calorie requirements, augmented by a dose or two of Endurance Amino to cover some of the amino acid requirements. It's certainly worth testing in your training!

With Endurance Amino, you're providing your body with a nice dose of multi-beneficial glutathione.

Now, in longer races (3+ hours or longer) the amino acids in Endurance Amino enhance the full-spectrum amino acid profile that naturally occurs from the protein component in Sustained Energy, Perpetuem, and Perpetuem Solids. However,

The Fast Lane

▶ With a combination of Endurance Amino and Sustained Energy or Perpetuem, you are getting more of some of the primary "during exercise" amino acids, without oversupplying the body with more amounts of amino acids that it may not really require.

with Endurance Amino we're only talking about a few specific amino acids—the three BCAAs, alanine, and glutathione (which is actually a tripeptide)—so you're not fully replacing the full-spectrum amino acid profile that occurs in Sustained Energy, Perpetuem, and Perpetuem Solids. For example, by going solely with Endurance Amino, you're not receiving any histidine, aspartic acid, or phenylalanine (among other amino acids), which have some "during exercise" benefits.

What you are getting with a combination of Endurance Amino and Sustained Energy, Perpetuem, or Perpetuem Solids is more of some of the primary "during exercise" amino acids, which is not a bad thing at all. In fact, we believe it's highly beneficial because you're providing the body with even greater amounts of some key "during exercise" amino acids without oversupplying the body with more amounts of amino acids that it may not really require. Plus, with Endurance Amino, you're providing your body with a nice dose of multi-beneficial glutathione.

Nolan Ming makes his way through the forest during The Kettle Moraine 100 in Wisconsin.
Photo : Rebekah Brummel

SUMMARY

The body is not equipped to replace "X" out with "X" or "near-X" back in, it knows this, and is very capable of "bridging the gap" between what it's losing calorie-wise and what it can accept in return from your fuel donation.

As you can see, there is a lot of information in this article to digest (no pun intended), but we're convinced that if you follow our recommendations you will no longer have to suffer with a number of performance-inhibiting problems—stomach issues included—that are the result of improper fueling.

When it comes to calorie replenishment, the amounts we recommend do not come anywhere near the "replace what you lose" figures that far too many so-called experts recommend. However, our recommendations more accurately reflect what your body can comfortably accept from you.

When considering your basic caloric needs, think complex carbohydrates such as the maltodextrin-based products, Hammer Gel and HEED, and—most of the time—a "complex carbohydrate + soy protein" fuel,

Sustained Energy, Perpetuem, or Perpeteum Solids for exercise over two hours.

Please remember that the most important point about our calorie intake recommendations is to customize them to your own personal needs. In your training log, make sure you include fueling data too. We give you "pretty close" numbers to start with, and you might end up with them also, but we don't offer them as a one-size-fits-all remedy. Besides body weight, your needs will vary with a number of factors such as fitness level, exercise intensity, weather, altitude, type of sport, and innate physiological differences.

RECOVERY

A crucial component for success

Professional triathlete Brendan Halpin in Tucson, Arizona. Photo : Vince Arnone

Often overlooked, always important

1. A workout places physical stress on your muscles and cardiovascular system. **Done right, this training creates just enough stress to cause an adaptive reaction that results in an increased level of fitness.**

2. **Training by itself, however, will not yield the results you want.** Remember, when you're done training, you're not done training . . . not until you've given your spent, depleted body the nutrition it needs to finish the job that your exercise or race has started. You need to supply your body with all of the needed nutrients so that it has the raw materials to build muscle, repair stressed tissues, and replace depleted energy and other nutrients.

3. **Effective recovery addresses three general areas:** carbohydrates for energy resupply, protein for muscle repair and rebuilding, and vitamins & minerals for micronutrient replenishment.

4. Timing is crucial to get the maximum benefit for the above physiological work. **Shortly after you finish your workout, you have a brief period of receptivity during which your body absorbs and metabolizes nutrients most efficiently.**

5. **In general, you want to get about**

10-20 grams of protein and 30-60 grams of complex carbs into your body within the first 30-60 minutes post-workout or race—the sooner the better. This is also an ideal time to consume vitamins, minerals, and antioxidants.

6. **In addition, to protect your general health in light of the stress of endurance training, you need specific supplements,** such as glutamine, that effectively bolster your immune system.

7. **Whey protein is the fastest absorbed of all proteins, with the highest levels of "recovery-specific" amino acids,** which makes it the best choice for recovery purposes.

8. **Heavy endurance training greatly increases your oxygen consumption and metabolism;** therefore, you need to incorporate a comprehensive panel of antioxidants into your recovery regimen.

9. **Recovery time is rehydration time, too.** A drink of Hammer Nutrition's Recoverite will provide the proper balance of carbohydrate and protein, along with plenty of fluid to wash down your recovery supplements.

Start reading the full article on page 76

INTRODUCTION

Training causes physical stress and depletion. Recovery is when adaptation to that stress occurs; it involves improvements not only in muscle performance, but also in glycogen storage. Hard training followed by timely, adequate nutritional replenishment increases your glycogen storage, as if your body is saying, "If there's another workout like this tomorrow, I better be prepared with a good supply of available fuel." If you feed your body correctly after a workout, you'll have that fuel, muscle glycogen, the next day.

This article answers questions about how to enhance your recovery, and it offers guidelines on what nutrients you need and how much of them to use. If you follow these guidelines, you'll give your body the support it requires to meet the demands of your next training session or race.

FULL ARTICLE

Athletes tend to focus on training and neglect recovery, specifically the critical step of refueling as soon as possible after each workout. We tend to think that a hard workout deserves a nice reward. Do you usually first go for a shower or relaxation after a hard workout? Are beer and pretzels your favored post-workout snack? If so, it's important to remember that a hard workout has left your body in a state of utter depletion and physiological vulnerability. However, it's also in a state of prime receptivity, ready to absorb nutrients. Taking those few extra minutes to properly refuel is one of the most important things that you can do to improve your race day results. In fact, properly refueling your body immediately after your training session is as important as anything you did in the actual workout.

You can really give yourself a major advantage come race day if you'll take the time to put some quality fuel into your body as soon as possible after all of your workouts. If you're at all serious about performing better in your racing and staying healthier, then take heed to this saying: "When you've finished training, you're still not finished with training!" Here's what I mean: You must attend as much to recovery as you do to active exercise if you expect to reap the benefits of hard training; how well you recover today will be a huge factor in how well you perform tomorrow. Exercise, done properly, creates enough stress on your muscles and cardiovascular system to instigate a rebuilding and strengthening program, but without causing big-time damage. Your body responds by adapting to the stress you placed upon it. Too much exercise at once leads to over-training syndrome. If you train within limits, but fail to supply your body with adequate fuel and nutrients, you get pretty much

Why is proper recovery so important?

- Your body will be able to store more and more of a premium, ready-to-use fuel known as muscle glycogen.

- You will strengthen, not weaken, your immune system.

- You will "kick start" the rebuilding of muscle tissue.

. . . .

Article continues here

much the same thing: over-use symptoms such as consistently sore muscles, increased susceptibility to infections, and fatigue.

Recovery includes many factors, including rest, stretching, muscle stimulation, and sleep, but we will limit our present discussion to the nutritional aspects. This article will cover the three essential nutritional areas of recovery: rehydration, the two macronutrients (carbohydrates and protein), and micronutrients (primarily antioxidants).

Rehydration

Technically, of course, water has no nutrient value, but it's essential for performance and recovery, and well worth a couple of paragraphs here. The normal course of recovery nutrition intake will meet most hydration needs, but it is possible for an athlete to suffer from chronic dehydration. In the article on hydration ("HYDRATION–What

you need to know" on page 22) we caution against excess fluid intake, a more common problem than dehydration, especially among the mass of recreational and fitness athletes. Top-level competitors, however, tend to under-hydrate during races.

As a rule of thumb, you want to finish a workout with no more than about 2% body weight loss, and certainly no weight gain. Weight loss in excess of 2% signals performance decline. For example, if you go out at 160 lbs (approx 72.5 kg) and return several hours later at 156 lbs (just under 71 kg), you're probably a bit dehydrated, but that would not be an unusual deficit after a hard workout or race. (Obviously, a steady, reliable scale is important here.) At a pint per pound (roughly 475 ml per kilogram), four pounds (nearly two kilograms) lost means you need to drink at least a good half-gallon (64 ounces, or just under two liters)

▶ The three essential nutritional
areas of recovery are:

Rehydration

The two macronutrients
(carbohydrates and protein)

Micronutrients
(primarily antioxidants)

▶ As a rule of thumb, you want
to finish a workout with no
more than about 2% body
weight loss, and certainly
no weight gain. Weight loss
in excess of 2% signals
performance decline.

▶ Carbohydrate replenishment
as soon as possible
after exercise, when the
body is most receptive
to carbohydrate uptake,
maximizes both glycogen
synthesis and storage.

**To paraphrase the late
Ed Burke, a well-known
nutritional scientist, on
recovery "The sooner
you do it, the better."**

of fluids in the next few hours. That's fairly
easy, and much of the fluid intake will
come in the normal course of nutritional
replenishment anyway.

Carbohydrate replenishment –
The sooner the better

Now let's consider carbohydrate
replenishment, the most obvious nutritional
issue caused by endurance exercise. When
you know the mechanism of carbohydrate
replenishment, you can very effectively
dial in your energy recovery program, so
let's briefly review your energy use and
restoration cycle.

When you begin a workout or race, the
primary fuel your body uses for the first
60-90 minutes or so is known as muscle
glycogen, a glucose polymer that contains
tens of thousands of glucose units arranged
in branched chains. As your stores of
muscle glycogen become depleted, your
body switches over to burning fat reserves
along with carbohydrates and protein
consumed during exercise. You've only
got a finite amount of this premium fuel,
muscle glycogen, but its importance can't
be overstated. In fact, several studies
have shown that the pre-exercise muscle
glycogen level is the most important energy
determinant for exercise performance.
Needless to say, to have a good race or
workout, you need to start with
a full load of muscle-stored
glycogen; athletes who have more
of this readily available fuel
in their bodies have a definite
advantage. The good news is that
you can substantially increase
your glycogen storage capacity
through the process of training
and replenishing. Here's how
your body does it: Along with
insulin, which regulates blood
sugar levels of ingested carbohydrates,
an enzyme known as glycogen synthase

converts carbohydrates from food into glycogen and stores it in muscle cells. This also drives the muscle repair and rebuilding process. However, to maximize the recovery process, you need to take advantage of glycogen synthase when it's most active. Carbohydrate replenishment as soon as possible after exercise, when the body is most receptive to carbohydrate uptake, maximizes both glycogen synthesis and storage. Glycogen synthesis from carbohydrate intake takes place most rapidly the first hour after exercise, remains fairly active perhaps another hour, and then occurs at diminished levels for up to six hours longer. Researchers at the University of Texas at Austin demonstrated that glycogen synthesis was highest when subjects were given carbohydrates immediately after exercise. Depletion followed immediately by carbohydrate intake yields the maximum glycogen resupply.

Complex carbohydrates versus simple sugars

The one time when your body isn't going to put up much of a fuss regarding complex carbohydrates versus simple sugars is right after a hard, glycogen-depleting workout. At this time, your body is in such dire need of replenishment that it'll accept just about anything. That said, complex carbohydrates still offer a distinct advantage over simple sugars, which is why

Eric Marquard blasts the bike leg at the 2010 Ironman Hawaii. Photo : ASI Photos

The Fast Lane

▶ Each American consumes about 133 pounds (60+ kg) of sugar annually. That's over 1/3 pound of sugar every day, 365 days a year!

▶ Simple sugars serve no purpose for recovery. Use only high glycemic, complex carbohydrates to optimally replenish glycogen stores.

▶ As soon as possible after you finish your workout, ideally within the first 30 minutes, consume 30-60 grams of high-quality, complex carbohydrates.

we strongly recommend using them. Here's why: Complex carbohydrates (such as the maltodextrin we use in Recoverite) and simple sugars (except fructose) have a high glycemic index (GI). This allows them to raise blood sugar levels and spike insulin rapidly, both desirable functions post-exercise. However, complex carbohydrates allow for a greater volume of calories to be absorbed compared to simple sugars. In other words, when you consume complex carbohydrates instead of simple sugars after exercise, your body is able to absorb more calories for conversion to glycogen without the increased potential for stomach distress that commonly occurs with simple sugar fuels.

Additionally, most of us already over-consume simple sugars from our daily diets. Numerous studies clearly show that sugar consumption in America is outrageously high. A report from the Berkeley Wellness Letter stated that each American consumes about 133 pounds (60+ kg) of sugar annually; that's over 1/3 pound sugar every day, 365 days a year! The USDA's "Dietary Assessment of Major Trends in U.S. Food Consumption, 1970-2005" (www.ers.usda.gov/Publications/EIB33/EIB33.pdf) illustrates the U.S. sugar/sweetener-consumption problem even more in stating, "In 2005, added sugars and sweeteners available for consumption totaled 142 pounds per person, up 19 percent since 1970."

It is abundantly clear that most-to-all of us are over-consuming sugar, and that excess sugar consumption is implicated in a number of health problems; for that reason alone their consumption should be extremely limited. Additionally, if they don't offer any specific post-workout benefits (which they don't), then why use them? (Note: Check out the many sugar-related articles on the Hammer Nutrition website—particularly the ones written by Nancy Appleton, Ph.D.—for more information on this important topic.)

The results are in!

• A less-fit athlete, or one who has not been refueling properly after exercise, has very limited muscle glycogen available, perhaps as little as 10-15 minutes worth.

• A fit athlete who has been consistently refueling his or her body with carbohydrates immediately after exercise can build up a glycogen supply that will last for up to 90 minutes of intense exercise. For instance, a well-trained 160 lb (72.5 kg) marathoner, packing some 2000 calories worth of premium fuel, can cover 18 miles in 90 minutes at a five min/mile pace. He'll need to consume some carbs to finish the race, but he's in good shape fuel-wise.

Which would you rather have when the gun goes off—15 minutes of on-board fuel or 90 minutes?

Article continues here

Bottom line: Simple sugars don't provide any benefits for general health or recovery. Use only high glycemic, complex carbohydrates (maltodextrins) to optimally replenish glycogen stores.

Important differences with athletic performance implications!

With what you've read so far, and after reading the information above, it should now be clear that by taking in ample amounts of carbohydrates immediately after training and continuing for the next few hours, you can get a head start on refueling your muscles after workouts. Additionally, consumption of carbohydrates will also tip the scales in the direction of protein synthesis instead of protein catabolism (breakdown). In other words, ample carbohydrates are essential in rebuilding muscle cells as well as restoring muscle glycogen. Studies suggest that the carbohydrate inflow gives the muscle cells the necessary fuel to begin the rebuilding process. Using the energy derived from carbohydrates, the muscles absorb amino acids from the bloodstream, helping initiate protein synthesis.

Carbohydrates also boost the production and release of insulin from the pancreas. Insulin is an anabolic (tissue-building) hormone that has a profound positive impact on protein synthesis in muscles, and it also tends to suppress protein breakdown. A University of Texas

▶ For optimum recovery, a mix of complex carbohydrates and protein is best.

▶ Whey protein is considered the ideal protein for recovery.

▶ Protein in your post-workout fuel provides these benefits:

- Raw materials to rebuild stressed muscles

- Enhanced glycogen storage

- Immune system maintenance

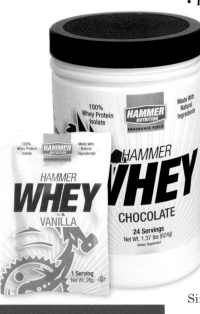

study found plasma insulin values three to eight times higher post-workout for subjects ingesting carbohydrates versus placebo.

Bottom line: For replenishing glycogen stores and aiding in the rebuilding of muscle tissue, quick replenishment of carbohydrates is a must. As soon as possible after you finish your workout, ideally within the first 30 minutes, consume 30-60 grams (the amount provided in 2-6 scoops of Recoverite) of high-quality complex carbohydrates.

Protein - Essential component for recovery

Carbohydrate intake promotes many aspects of post-exercise recovery, but it can't do the job alone; you need protein as well. Protein in your post-workout fuel provides these benefits:

• **Raw materials to rebuild stressed muscles** – Whey protein is the premier protein source of the three branched chain amino acids (BCAAs – leucine, isoleucine, valine) used for muscle tissue repair.

• **Enhanced glycogen storage** – Numerous studies have shown that the consumption of carbohydrates plus protein, versus carbohydrates alone, is a superior way to maximize post-exercise muscle glycogen synthesis.

• **Immune system maintenance** – We strongly recommend whey protein, with its high levels of amino acids that spur glutathione production (see below).

Whey is the superior protein source for recovery

A standard known as Biological Value (BV) is an accurate indicator of biological activity of protein, a scale used to determine the percentage of a given nutrient that the body utilizes. Simply put, BV refers to how well and how quickly your body can actually use the protein that you consume.

Of all protein sources, whey has the highest BV, with whey protein isolate (the purest form of whey protein) having an outstanding rating of 154, and whey protein concentrate having a 104 rating. Egg protein also has an outstanding BV, with whole eggs rating 100 and egg whites (albumin) rated at 88. With a 49 rating, soy protein ranks far below whey protein, making it a less desirable choice for recovery. (When the BV system was introduced, eggs had the highest known BV and thus were given a value of 100. Whey proteins came to researchers' attention later, and they rang up even higher scores. The 154 BV of whey protein isolate and the 104 BV of whey concentrate are in comparison with the original BV benchmark, whole eggs.)

Other standards that evaluate protein quality/effect also show whey to be a superb protein source.

One of these methods, the Protein Efficiency Ratio (PER), while it admittedly has limited applications for humans (PER measures the weight gain of experimental growing rats when being fed the test protein), still shows that whey protein ranks the highest, with a rating of 3.6 (soy protein has a rating of 2.1).

Another protein measurement is the Protein Digestibility Corrected Amino Acid Score (PDCAAS). Nutritionists who disqualify the PER method for classifying protein quality (because it only references the amino acid requirements for lab rats) often will use the PDCAAS method for evaluating human protein requirements. According to this method, which utilizes an amino acid requirement profile derived from human subjects, an ideal protein is one that meets all of the essential amino acid requirements of humans. An ideal protein receives a rating of 1.0. Three protein sources—whey, soy,

Joe Neczek celebrates his 2nd place age group medal with his children at the 2010 Wisconsin Triterium Triathlon. Photo : Angie Neczek

One very important point about whey protein: make sure you use whey protein isolate, not whey protein concentrate. Whey protein isolate is virtually lactose and fat free; many lactose-intolerant people can still use whey protein isolate because it contains only a minuscule amount of lactose. Also, whey isolate checks in at a sturdy 90-97+% protein, whereas whey concentrate contains only 70-80% protein (and, unfortunately, oftentimes less). Simply put, whey protein isolate is a purer protein, and the best protein you can put into your body after a hard workout.

Hammer Whey and the whey protein used in Recoverite come from cows that are not treated with antibiotics. Every load that is taken into the plant for processing is tested for antibiotics and rejected if it contains any. The end product is a pure, undenatured whey protein isolate of the highest quality. It is 98% pure, virtually fat free, and carbohydrate-free. The whey protein isolate in Hammer Whey and Recoverite delivers rich immune-enhancing beta-lactoalbumins and alpha-lactalbumins. Hammer Whey has a unique profile of highly bioavailable protein with immune factors, potent branched chain amino acids (BCAAs), lactoferrin, and immunoglobulins. Independent laboratory tests show the PDCAAS (Protein Digestibility Corrected Amino Acid Score) for the whey protein isolate in Hammer Whey and Recoverite is a whopping 1.14, a score that exceeds all of those reported for egg, milk, caseinates, and soy protein.

Glutathione: The key to optimal immune system support & recovery

Glutathione is a tripeptide consisting of the amino acids glutamic acid, cysteine, and glycine. It is one of the three endogenous (naturally occurring in the

The Fast Lane

▶ Make sure that you use whey protein isolate, not whey protein concentrate. Whey protein isolate is virtually lactose and fat free; many lactose-intolerant people can still use whey protein isolate because it contains only a minuscule amount of lactose.

Whey vs. Soy
Glutathione and amino acid comparisons

Table A
Hammer Whey/Recoverite vs. Hammer Soy

A comparison for glutathione production (approximate amounts per gram of protein)

Amino Acid	Whey Isolate	Soy
Cysteine	33 mg	9 mg
Methionine	17 mg	9 mg
Glutamic Acid	103 mg	138 mg
Glutamine	333 mg	10.5 mg

Table B
Hammer Whey/Recoverite vs. Hammer Soy

A comparison (approximate amounts per gram of protein) of BCAAs (branched chain amino acids)

Amino Acid	Whey Isolate	Soy
Leucine	100 mg	59 mg
Isoleucine	51 mg	35 mg
Valine	36 mg	36 mg

Article continues here

body) antioxidants, the other two being catalase and superoxide dismutase. Many researchers rate glutathione as the number one antioxidant. Ward Dean, MD, a leading nutritional scientist, in his brilliant article "Glutathione: Life-Extending 'Master Antioxidant," addresses the importance of glutathione, stating that "Glutathione is present in nearly all living cells, and without it they can't survive . . . glutathione has major effects on health at the molecular, cellular, and organ levels."

One of the most important steps we can take to improve our recovery is to enhance/optimize body levels of this important antioxidant, and one of the best ways to do that is by consuming whey protein. Whey protein contains excellent levels of all three of the amino acids that comprise glutathione, as well as high levels of the sulfur-containing amino acids methionine and cysteine. These two amino acids are particularly important for proper immune system function and the body's production of glutathione. In addition, the amino acid glutamine has also been shown to help raise glutathione levels (both Hammer Nutrition whey protein products, Hammer Whey and Recoverite, contain high amounts of glutamine). See Table A above.

Bottom line: Adequate glutathione in the body will enhance your recovery and support optimal health.

Branched Chain Amino Acids (BCAAs) – Essential for muscle repair

Of the nearly two dozen different amino acids required by humans, nine are classified as essential because they cannot be synthesized by the body and must be derived from external food sources. Among these nine essential amino acids are the branched chain amino acids leucine, isoleucine, and valine. The term "branched chain" refers to the molecular structure of these particular amino acids. Up to 75% of the body's muscle tissue is composed of these three amino acids, and they are directly involved in the tissue repair process. BCAAs are present in all protein-containing foods, with whey protein being the best source. See Table B on page 85.

Bottom line: Soy protein is certainly an excellent protein source for a variety of health benefits. However, when it comes to enhancing recovery between workouts—maximizing glycogen synthesis, supporting immune system function, and rebuilding lean muscle tissue—you simply won't find a better protein source than whey protein isolate. After your workouts, consume 10-30 grams of protein, preferably whey isolate, along with your complex carbohydrates. For more information about protein, see the article "PROTEIN–Why it's important for endurance athletes."*

Recoverite - The perfect carb/protein product

If you've read this far, you might be asking yourself, "That's all fine in theory, but how in the world do I get all those high quality carbohydrates and protein into my body after a workout?" Good question, and we have a good answer, because we've formulated a premier recovery-specific product called Recoverite. Recoverite is the easy way to take care of crucial recovery needs for serious

The Fast Lane

▶ Of the nearly two dozen different amino acids required by humans, nine are classified as essential because they cannot be synthesized by the body and must be derived from external food sources.

▶ Recoverite is the easy way to take care of crucial recovey needs for serious endurance athletes, providing high-quality complex carbohydrates and whey protein isolate.

▶ Each serving of Recoverite also supplies a potent, recovery-boosting three grams of l-glutamine.

* Article Reference
"PROTEIN–Why it's important for endurance athletes"
Page 130

endurance athletes, providing the high-quality complex carbohydrates and whey protein isolate you need. Additionally, Recoverite supplies a generous amount of glutamine, a couple of other recovery-specific micronutrients, and a full-spectrum electrolyte profile. It's the ideal post-workout fuel.

Why a 3:1 carbohydrate to protein ratio?

As mentioned earlier in the article, timely post-workout carbohydrate and protein replenishment helps optimize glycogen synthesis and rebuild muscle tissue. While other products use a 4:1 ratio of carbohydrates to protein, Recoverite supplies the two components in a 3:1 ratio, which we believe is the ideal ratio for enhanced recovery. Dr. Bill Misner explains:

> Research supports the concept for utilizing four parts carbohydrate to one part protein during the [brief] window-of-opportunity in order to exogenously impact lean muscle mass growth and glycogen restorage. Shortly after Ivy and Burke and several others specified results with a 4:1 ratio, a patented product was then marketed. Another research paper using elderly subjects in strength exercise (weights) found conclusively that when these subjects lifted weights three days per week and consumed one part carbohydrate to one part protein, they positively achieved lean muscle mass growth gains. This later study skews the conclusion of the former, calling for the question of what carbohydrate

to protein ratio best supports lean muscle mass growth and glycogen restorage post-depletion workout. In other words, research is inconclusively leaning toward the 4:1 ratio, but has not excluded the 3:1 or 5:1 ratios, due to not having studied them as much as the patented 4:1 ratio. This leaves me with the opinion that as far as conclusive research data goes, the jury is still out, waiting for more papers to be published on other ratio values.

An endurance exercise session lasting more than three hours depletes muscle glycogen and likely cannibalizes around 50-60 grams of lean muscle proteins, and probably around 500-600 grams of glycogen, which should be replaced. The total dietary replacement ratio then is at least 10:1 carbohydrates

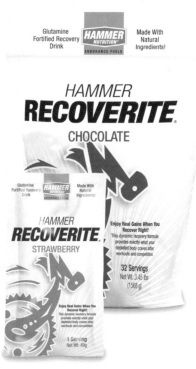

The Fast Lane

▶ For rebuilding lean muscle tissue and immune system support, whey protein isolate has no peer; it's simply the purest form of whey protein available.

▶ The 3:1 carbohydrate to protein post-exercise protocol is rational for the endurance athlete, especially if lean muscle mass recovery is the objective.

to protein. Since the glycogen synthase enzyme released during glycogen depletion has a short half-life effective for 90-120 minutes, but most effectively available at 30 minutes post-exercise, it behooves us (according to Colgan, Costill, Noakes, Hawley, Ivy, etc.) to drive replacement proteins on the insulin-glycogen synthase "train" for effective maximal replacement. If you try to replace all of the glycogen in one or two meals, spaced an hour apart with all the protein, too much carbohydrate in one meal will produce excess adipose fatty acid storage. Cutting the carbs down to small doses will produce the insulin and provide maximum storage rates for the protein fraction delivery into the muscle cell for the lean muscle mass rebuilding process.

The 3:1 carbohydrate to protein post-exercise protocol is rational for the endurance athlete, especially if lean muscle mass recovery is the objective. Adding one more part carbohydrate raises the carbohydrate component (to 4:1) and may be beneficial for athletes who are free from carbohydrate-induced fat weight. Of the two ratios—3:1 or 4:1—the lower-carb Recoverite formula appears to be favorable for lean muscle gain than the patented 4:1 higher carb formula. Altering the formula in any direction toward more protein or more carbohydrate should be monitored by fat weight gain and lean muscle mass gain accordingly.

Since we've noted research that showed positive lean muscle mass growth in older subjects using a 1:1 carbohydrate to protein recovery formula for, our opinion is that the lower carbohydrate version [3:1 ratio] is superior to the higher carbohydrate version.

Protein and ancillary nutrients

Regarding protein, Recoverite contains only

whey protein isolate, which we discussed earlier. For rebuilding lean muscle tissue and immune system support, whey protein isolate has no peer; it's simply the purest form of whey protein available. In addition, each serving of Recoverite also supplies a potent, recovery-boosting three grams of l-glutamine. The benefits of l-glutamine are hard to overstate. Among other things, it plays a crucial role in preserving and rebuilding lean tissue as well as supporting the immune system following intense exercise. In addition, l-glutamine is vital for gastrointestinal health.

Recoverite also supplies two other recovery-enhancing nutrients—chromium polynicotinate and l-carnosine.

The trace mineral chromium helps regulate carbohydrate metabolism. This has profound effects on athletic performance, especially recovery. Studies suggest that athletes who consume chromium polynicotinate (along with ample carbohydrates) within two hours of completion of exercise will experience a 300% increase in the rate of glycogen synthesis compared to no supplementation. In addition to the chromium provided in a serving of Recoverite, an additional 200 mcg of ChromeMate™ is an excellent recovery-boosting strategy.

L-carnosine, also known simply as carnosine, is one of the most versatile and beneficial nutrients that you can put in your body. During exercise it's a great lactic acid buffer, and afterwards it continues to offer antioxidant and antiglycation benefits.

The Fast Lane

▶ To enhance recovery, it's important to replenish basic vitamins and minerals depleted during exercise.

▶ To completely replenish vitamins and minerals lost during exercise, use a product that provides adequate amounts of the full spectrum of necessary vitamins and minerals like Premium Insurance Caps.

▶ Our bodies need antioxidants to protect us from the damaging effects of free radicals.

Antiglycation is a process that may play a substantial role in preventing age-related physiological decline. One theory of aging focuses on the damage done to the cells by free radicals, which antioxidants help neutralize. Another theory of aging points to irreversible damage to the body's proteins caused by a process called glycation. A simple definition of glycation is the cross-linking of proteins and sugars to form nonfunctioning structures in the body. Glycation is cited as an underlying cause of age-related problems including neurologic (brain), vascular (circulatory), and ocular (eye) disorders. Carnosine has been shown to help prevent glycation.

Recoverite also contains a full-spectrum electrolyte profile, which helps replenish depleted essential electrolytes.

Bottom line: Recoverite provides unsurpassed nutritional support to ensure that you obtain the maximum value from your workouts and complete recovery after each training session and race.

Micronutrient replenishment

To enhance recovery, it's important to replenish basic vitamins and minerals depleted during exercise. Additionally, it's extremely important to provide the body with a variety of antioxidants. You may have noticed that we have not mentioned Recoverite's vitamin profile. That's because it contains none. Yes, vitamins are indeed important in recovery, but most, if not all, recovery products contain only a limited number of vitamins and/or insignificant amounts of whatever vitamins they do provide. To completely replenish vitamins and minerals lost during exercise, use a product that provides adequate amounts of the full spectrum of necessary vitamins and minerals. For satisfying this important aspect of recovery, Premium Insurance Caps, a potent, complete vitamin/mineral

Your antioxidant arsenal

Recoverite

Cysteine*, Methionine*, Glutamic Acid*, Glutamine*, Carnosine

Premium Insurance Caps

Beta Carotene, Vitamin C*, Vitamin E, Zinc, Selenium*, Manganese

Race Caps Supreme

Coenzyme Q10, Idebenone, Vitamin E, Trimethylglycine

Mito Caps

Vitamin C (as ascorbyl palmitate)*, Vitamin E, Acetyl l-carnitine, R-alpha Lipoic Acid*, DMAE (Dimethylaminoethanol), PABA (Para Amino Benzoic Acid)

AO Booster

Gamma E Tocopherol Complex, Tocomin® Full-Spectrum Natural Tocotrienol Complex, Lutein, Astaxanthin

Super Antioxidant

Enteric Coated Super Oxide Dismutase, Grape Seed Extract*, L-Glutathione*, Ginkgo biloba, Gotu kola, Vinpocetine

*Glutathione precursors and/or glutathione boosting nutrients

. . . .

Article continues here

supplement, is ideal.

Bottom line: While recovery drinks may provide some of the basic vitamins and minerals, they're either lacking in certain ones and/or contain only token amounts. To fulfill your basic vitamin/mineral requirements more completely, don't rely on what a recovery drink provides; use Premium Insurance Caps.

Antioxidants - Your body's protection against free radicals

Our bodies need antioxidants to protect us from the damaging effects of free radicals. Free radicals (of which there are several types) are unstable atoms or molecules, usually of oxygen, containing at least one unpaired electron. Left unchecked, free radicals seek out and literally steal electrons from whole atoms or molecules, creating a destructive chain reaction. Excess free radicals, in the words of one nutritional scientist, "are capable of damaging virtually any biomolecule, including proteins, sugars, fatty acids, and nucleic acids."

Dr. Bill Misner writes: *Oxygen has the capacity to be both friend and foe. When energy fuels are metabolized in the presence of O2, 5% of them create molecules that contain an odd number of electrons. If free radicals are not neutralized immediately by on-site antioxidant body stores, tissue damage occurs to absolutely every cell membrane touched by these imbalanced molecular wrecking machines. Some theorize that soreness and stiffness result because*

91

free radicals and waste metabolites build up during either prolonged or intense exercise. The more volume oxygen that passes into our physiology for energy fuel metabolism, the more increased free radical-fatigue symptoms may be experienced.

▶ Excellent antioxidant-rich foods include:

Almonds	Pecans
Apples	Pineapples
Apricots	Pistachios
Artichokes	Plums
Avocados	Radishes
Beets	Raspberries
Bell peppers	Spinach
Blackberries	Squash
Blueberries	Strawberries
Broccoli	Tomatoes
Cabbage	Walnuts
Cantaloupe	
Carrots	
Cashews	
Cauliflower	
Citrus fruits	
Grapefruit	
Grapes	
Mangoes	
Peaches	

These words should sound the alarm bells loud and clear, because as an athlete you consume huge amounts of oxygen and metabolize far greater amounts of calories than a sedentary person does. This means that you're generating free radicals on the order of 12-20 times more than non-athletes! During periods of peak training and racing stress, free radical production increases even more. While the benefits of exercise far outweigh the potential negatives caused by free radicals, excess free radical production and accumulation, if not properly resolved, may very well be the endurance athlete's worst foe. The human body can oxidize and decay, like rusting steel, from excess free radical production. Not only can this negate everything that you've worked so hard to achieve in your training, but it can also result in severe consequences to your overall health.

Clearly, the necessity of neutralizing excess free radicals cannot be overstated, which is why we recommend supplementation with a variety of antioxidants. On the following pages we list a number of antioxidant-rich Hammer Nutrition products. More detailed information, along with dosage suggestions, can be found in the supplement to this book, *The Hammer Nutrition Fuels & Supplements–Everything you need to know.* For now these are the salient points to keep in mind:

• Antioxidants are a group of micronutrients that are desperately needed post-workout.

• You need a wide spectrum of antioxidants because prolonged exercise produces many different types of free radicals. Each antioxidant targets different free radicals, so don't make the mistake of thinking that any one antioxidant, say vitamin E, will protect you from all of the ravages of free radical production.

• Consuming antioxidant-rich foods and taking antioxidant supplements throughout the day—targeting primary intake post-workout—is an ideal way to support enhanced immune system health.

Putting it all together – Recovery nutrition recommendations

After extensive training sessions or races, in addition to Recoverite or Hammer Whey + carbohydrates, we recommend the following supplements.

▶ **Premium Insurance Caps** – to help replenish the body's stores of essential vitamins and minerals, including some vital antioxidants. There's no doubt that your body will have depleted its stores of vitamins and minerals, and quick replenishment will enhance recovery and protect the immune system. Several capsules also provide a substantial dose of chromium polynicotinate, which, as mentioned earlier, is a vital micronutrient involved

in the glycogen resupply process. After exceptionally difficult and/ or lengthy workouts, an additional 200mcg capsule of ChromeMate™ should also be considered.

▶ **Race Caps Supreme** – for its three very powerful antioxidants – Coenzyme Q10, idebenone, and vitamin E. Not only does it support enhanced energy production during exercise (from those nutrients plus other key substrates), it also supports enhanced recovery after your workouts. Additionally, all three nutrients play key roles in maintaining optimal cardiovascular health.

▶ **Mito Caps** – arguably the most potent supplement you can take for recovery and overall health. The combination of acetyl l-carnitine (ALC) and r-alpha lipoic acid (R-ALA) has many

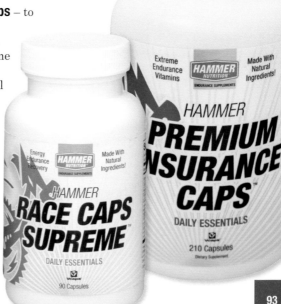

▶ Each athlete must design an individualized supplement program to meet his or her particular bodily demands and performance goals.

▶ If you want to reap the benefits out of all the time and energy you put into your training, as soon as possible after you finish your workout—ideally within the first 30-60 minutes

extraordinary benefits; to list them all would fill a book. These two powerful nutrients provide immune system support, lean muscle tissue preservation via decreased levels of excess cortisol, and optimal functioning of the mitochondria, your body's energy producing "furnaces." The R-ALA component is especially beneficial in that it extends the usable life of antioxidants such as vitamin C, vitamin E, and glutathione.

▶ **AO Booster** – If there were only one or two types of free radicals negatively affecting our bodies, we'd be able to get by with one, maybe two, antioxidants such as vitamin C and vitamin E. The truth, however, is that there are a number of free radicals, both water-soluble and fat-soluble, which is why a wide variety of antioxidants is necessary. With AO Booster you have an arsenal of powerful fat-soluble antioxidants to provide even more immune system-boosting power to the water-soluble ones provided in the three previously-mentioned products and Super Antioxidant (discussed next). In addition, with AO Booster you'll also notice benefits for your eyes and skin, as well as reduced muscle soreness and inflammation.

▶ **Super Antioxidant** – perhaps the strongest non-vitamin antioxidant formula available. As mentioned earlier, because athletes exchange several hundred times more oxygen than sedentary people do, free radical production is a certainty. Left unchecked, free radicals can damage cell membranes, suppress the immune system, and delay recovery. To protect the body's cells and to promote accelerated recovery, sufficient antioxidant intake is critical. Super Antioxidant perfectly complements the antioxidants found in the earlier-mentioned four products. In addition, several of the nutrients in the product provide additional recovery-enhancing benefits via their effects on increasing circulation. Lastly, the grape seed extract component in Super Antioxidant, in addition to providing substantial free radical-neutralizing benefits, is believed to aid in strengthening and repairing connective tissue while also providing anti-inflammation support.

▶ **Xobaline** – for its influence on the resynthesis of RNA, the basis for cellular reproduction. Research suggests that improving RNA "status" within the body results in gains in lean muscle mass, increased mitochondrial resynthesis, and other benefits. When this occurs, the athlete may expect increased energy, improved metabolism, and enhanced recovery after exercise. In addition, the folic acid/vitamin B12 combination is vital for healthy red blood cell production and cardiovascular health, via the reduction of elevated homocysteine levels.

SUMMARY

How well you recover today greatly determines how well you'll perform tomorrow.

The fact is that athletes who attend to the recovery process as much as they do to active training have a distinct advantage over athletes who disregard or neglect it. Therefore, if you want to reap the benefits out of all the time and energy you put into your training, as soon as possible after you finish your workout—ideally within the first 30-60 minutes—it's crucial for you to replenish your body with adequate amounts of complex carbohydrates, whey protein isolate, and supplementary vitamins, minerals, and a wide variety of antioxidants.

If you will follow these simple recommendations consistently, you will unquestionably see noticeable improvements in the quality of your workouts as well as better race results. Additionally, via the nutritional support you're providing your body, your overall health will benefit as well.

PROPER FUELING

▶ Pre-workout & race suggestions

Shaun Radley at the Firecracker 50. He completed the day with an 11th place age-group finish. Photo : Mountain Moon Photography - Annette Hayden

What to eat and when

1. The title is somewhat of a misnomer, because you don't really need a full-fledged meal before a workout or race; just a snack to top off your liver glycogen. **Your muscle glycogen, the first fuel recruited when exercise begins, does not deplete overnight.**

2. You don't need a big meal. You don't need much protein, if any. You don't need fiber. You need little, if any fat, and you want zero saturated fat. **This isn't the time for a fully-balanced, healthy meal. You primarily want easy to digest complex carbs.**

3. **Whatever you eat, finish it at least three hours before commencing exercise to allow adequate time for digestion, absorption, and your blood glucose regulation system to normalize.**

4. **Pre-exercise hunger is not a sign of depleted glycogen; you can begin a workout or race when hungry. Once you get going, the hunger will stop.** You do, however, want a full load of muscle glycogen, and that only comes from months of endurance training and proper recovery nutrition. You will not gain anything (except weight) by carbo-loading before a race.

5. A good pre-exercise snack might consist of a serving or two of Hammer Gel, a serving of Sustained Energy or Perpetuem, a bagel, a baked potato, or some combination of these.

Start reading the full article on page 98

INTRODUCTION

Over the past eleven+ years, many of the athletes I've worked with have been reluctant to adopt these plans—until they actually try them. Then they're convinced by their improved performance, and they never go back to the conventional advice. The recommendations in this article may seem counterintuitive, but physiologically speaking, they make perfect sense. Adopt and use them consistently in your training and watch your performance soar!

FULL ARTICLE

How many times have you had a bite (or more) from an energy bar, taken a swig (or more) from an energy drink, or eaten a meal just an hour or two before starting a lengthy workout or taking your position at the starting line of a long distance race? Big mistake! Eating this soon before prolonged exercise is actually counterproductive and will hurt your performance. In the sometimes confusing world of sports supplementation and fueling,

Equally as important as what you eat is when you eat your pre-exercise meal.

pre-exercise food/fuel consumption generates arguably the greatest confusion, and many athletes have paid a hefty performance price for their misinformation. But really, there's no insider secret regarding what to do for a pre-workout/race meal, just some effective strategies and guidelines. You need to know what to eat, how much, and most importantly, when. You also need to know a bit about glycogen storage, depletion, and resupply, and how to

use that knowledge at the practical level. This article supplies all of the information you need, and I've also included some suggested meals, equally appropriate for workouts as well as competition.

The goal of pre-exercise calorie consumption

Assuming that your workout or race starts in the morning, the purpose of your pre-race meal is to top off liver glycogen stores, which your body has expended during your night of sleep. Muscle glycogen, the first fuel recruited when exercise commences, remains intact overnight. If you had a proper recovery meal after your last workout, you'll have a full load of muscle glycogen on board, which constitutes about 80% of your total glycogen stores. If you didn't resupply with complex carbs and protein after your last workout, there's nothing you can do about it now; in fact, you'll only hurt yourself by trying. To repeat: during sleep, your liver-stored glycogen maintains a proper blood glucose level; you expend nary a calorie of your muscle glycogen. You might wake up feeling hungry, and I'll

Pre-workout/race meal
Fulfill the carbohydrate+protein recommendation

Sustained Energy which contains both complex carbohydrates and soy protein

Perpetuem, which contains complex carbohydrates, soy protein, and a small donation of healthy fats

A combination of Sustained Energy + Hammer Gel or HEED

Article continues here

discuss that issue later, but you'll have a full supply of muscle-stored glycogen. Your stomach might be saying, "I'm hungry," but your muscles are saying, "Hey, we're good to go!"

With only your liver-stored glycogen to top off, you want a light pre-race nutrition meal. Sports nutrition expert Bill Misner, Ph.D., advises that a pre-workout/race meal should be "an easily digested, high complex carbohydrate meal of between 200-400 calories with a minimum of fiber, simple sugar, and fat." That's hardly what most folks would call a meal, but in terms of pre-exercise fueling, it's meal enough. According to Dr. Misner, fat slows digestion and has no positive influence on fuels metabolized during an event. He further states that a meal high in fiber may "create the call for an unscheduled and undesirable bathroom break in the middle or near the end of the event."

Complex carbohydrates & protein

One study found that athletes who drank a meal consisting of both carbohydrates and a small amount of protein had better performances than when they consumed only an all-carbohydrate sports drink.

If you do feel the need for solid food instead of a liquid fuel meal, choose high starch foods such as skinless potatoes, bananas, rice, pasta, plain bagels, low fat active culture yogurt, tapioca, and low fiber hot cereals.

The key – Allow three hours or more!

Equally as important as what you eat is when you eat your pre-exercise meal. Authorities such as Dr. Misner, Dr. Michael Colgan, and Dr. David Costill all agree that the pre-race meal should be eaten 3-4 hours prior to the event. Dr. Misner suggests the athlete "leave three hours minimum to digest foods eaten at breakfast. After breakfast, drink 10-12 ounces of fluid each hour up to 30 minutes prior to the start (24-30 ounces total fluid intake)." Note: other acceptable pre-race fluid intake suggestions can be found in the article "HYDRATION–What you need to know" on page 22.

Three hours allows enough time for your body to fully process the meal. Colgan says it's the digestion time necessary to avoid intestinal distress. Costill's landmark study [Costill DL. Carbohydrates for exercise. Dietary demand for optimal performance. Int J Sports 1988;9:1-18] shows that complex carbohydrates consumed 3-4 hours prior to exercise raise blood glucose and improve performance. But it's Misner's argument that has proved most compelling to me.

Dr. Misner's rationale – It's all in the timing

▶ You must complete your pre-workout/race fueling three or more hours prior to the start to allow adequate time for insulin and blood glucose to normalize.

▶ What to do if you wake up very hungry and feel the need to eat before a workout or race:

- Just start anyway, realizing that hunger is not a performance inhibitor

- If you must, consume 100-200 calories five minutes before start time

If you consume high glycemic carbohydrates such as simple sugars (or even the preferred complex carbohydrates such as starches and maltodextrins) within three hours of exercise, you can expect the following, with possible negative effects on performance:

1. Rapidly elevated blood sugar causes excess insulin release, leading to hypoglycemia, an abnormally low level of glucose in the blood.

2. High insulin levels inhibit lipid mobilization during aerobic exercise, which means reduced fats-to-fuels conversion. Our ability to utilize stored fatty acids as energy largely determines our performance, which is why we can continue to exercise when our caloric intake falls far below our energy expenditure. We want to enhance, not impede, our stored fat utilization pathways.

3. A high insulin level will induce blood sugar into muscle cells, which increases the rate of carbohydrate metabolism, hence rapid carbohydrate fuel depletion. In simple terms: high insulin means faster muscle glycogen depletion.

You must complete your pre-workout/race fueling three or more hours prior to the start to allow adequate time for insulin and blood glucose to normalize. After three hours, hormonal balance is restored, and you won't be at risk for increased glycogen depletion. Eating within three hours of a training session or race promotes faster release/depletion of both liver and muscle glycogen and inhibits fat utilization. The combination of accelerated glycogen depletion and disruption of your primary long-distance fuel availability can devastate your performance.

But I'm hungry!

Recall that I mentioned earlier that muscle glycogen, the main fuel recruited for the first 60-90 minutes of exercise, remains unaffected by a night-long fast. When you awaken in the morning, you haven't lost your primary fuel supply, and can't add to it by eating within an hour or two of exercise. That's absolutely correct, and believe it or not, being hungry before an event won't inhibit performance.

However, hard-training athletes often do wake up very hungry and feel they need to eat something before their workout or race. This is especially true for half and full iron-distance triathletes, who start very early in the morning in the water, swimming for up to an hour or more, which makes consuming food impossible.

What to do? Try either of the following suggestions to help with this problem:

1. Just start anyway, realizing that hunger is not a performance inhibitor, and begin fueling shortly after you start, when you get into a comfortable rhythm. The hunger sensation will diminish almost as soon as you begin to exercise, and you'll actually be benefiting, not hurting, your performance by following this procedure. You can safely use Sustained Energy, Perpetuem, HEED, or Hammer Gel, or any combination thereof, as soon as you want after exercise commences. For details regarding appropriate amounts,

Shane Ellis rockets around the Encino Velodrome in Encino, California.
Photo : David Paul Green, Monteverdi Creative

The Fast Lane

▶ When you're engaged in training sessions or races in the 90-minute or shorter range, fasting three hours prior to the start is not necessary.

▶ If you're a fit athlete, you have approximately 60-90 minutes of stored muscle glycogen available.

▶ When you consume calories within three hours of a race you will accelerate muscle glycogen utilization.

* Article Reference
  "CALORIC INTAKE–
  Proper amounts during
  endurance exercise"
  Page 54

please refer to the article "CALORIC INTAKE–Proper amounts during endurance exercise."*

2. If you feel that you absolutely must eat, consume 100-200 calories about five minutes before start time. By the time these calories are digested and blood sugar levels are elevated, you'll be well into your workout or race, and glycogen depletion will not be negatively affected. In this regard, good choices are one or two servings of Hammer Gel or a generous drink from a premixed bottle of Sustained Energy or Perpetuem. This strategy is especially appropriate for triathletes who will hit the water first and not have a chance to replenish calories right away. Small amounts of nutrient-dense fuels, such as those named above, go a long way to stanching hunger pangs.

Are there any exceptions to the three-hour rule?

When you're engaged in training sessions or races in the 90-minute range or shorter (personally, I prefer an hour limit), fasting three hours prior to the start is not necessary. Consuming some easily digested calories an hour or two prior to the start will not negatively affect performance, and may actually enhance it. Here's why:

As we've discussed earlier, when you consume calories sooner than three hours prior to the start of a workout or race, you accelerate the rate at which your body burns its finite amounts of muscle glycogen stores. In events lasting longer than 60-90 minutes, refraining from calorie consumption for the three-hour period prior to the start is crucial because you want to preserve your glycogen stores, not accelerate their depletion. Your body has a limited supply of this premium fuel so if your workout or race goes beyond the 60-90 minute mark, you don't want to do

Sleep or eat?

Q: Should I get up during the wee hours of the morning just to get in a meal three hours before my race or workout?

A: NO—rest will help you more. Much restorative physiology occurs during sleep, so don't sacrifice sleep just to eat. If you're a fit athlete, one who has been replenishing carbohydrates immediately after each exercise session, you have approximately 60-90 minutes of muscle glycogen, your premium fuel, available. As long as you begin fueling shortly after the workout or race begins, perhaps 10-20 minutes after the start, your performance will not be affected negatively. Topping off liver glycogen stores is always a good idea, but not at the expense of sacrificing sleep, and certainly not at the expense of depleting muscle glycogen stores too quickly (by eating too soon before exercise).

Article continues here

anything that will accelerate muscle glycogen utilization. However, when you consume calories within three hours of a race, that's exactly what will happen; you'll increase the rate at which your glycogen is burned.

During shorter distance races, however, accelerated rates of glycogen depletion/utilization are not problematic. You don't need the calories for energy, but the presence of carbohydrates will elevate glycogen utilization. In a short race, that's what you want.

Dr. Misner explains that prior to shorter-duration bouts of exercise, ". . . consuming a few easily digested carbohydrates [such as a serving or two of HEED or Hammer Gel] will advance performance, because carbohydrates consumed prior to exercise make the body super-expend its glycogen stores like a flood gate wide open." In other words, if you eat something 1-2 hours prior to the start of a short-duration training session or race, thus causing the insulin "flood gates" to open, yes, you will be depleting your glycogen stores at maximum rates. However, at this distance it's a beneficial effect, as glycogen depletion is not an issue when the workout or race is over within at the most 90 minutes.

This advice assumes that you have been effectively refueling your body after each workout, as this is the primary way to increase muscle glycogen (see the article

Our pre-exercise fueling recommendations

- Eat 200-400 calories at least three hours before exercise.

- Focus on complex carbs, starches, and a little protein.

- Avoid high fiber, simple sugars, and high fat (especially saturated fat).

- If you must, consume a small amount of your supplemental fuel (Hammer Gel, etc.) about five minutes before exercise.

- Make sure that you re-supply your muscle glycogen by eating a good recovery meal after your workouts.

Any of the pre-exercise meal suggestions below will keep you in the preferred 200-400 calorie range:

- Three scoops of Sustained Energy
- Two scoops of Sustained Energy flavored with one serving of Hammer Gel or one scoop of HEED
- Two to three servings of Hammer Gel or two to three scoops of HEED fortified with one scoop of Sustained Energy
- Two to two and a half scoops of Perpetuem

- One white flour bagel and a half cup of active yogurt
- A banana and a cup of active yogurt
- Cream of Rice, sweetened with a serving of Hammer Gel
- One soy protein-enhanced pancake, sweetened with a serving of Hammer Gel
- Half of a skinless baked potato with a half cup of plain active yogurt

Article continues here

"RECOVERY–A crucial component of athletic success" for details)*.

* Article Reference
"RECOVERY–A crucial component of athletic success"
Page 74

Bottom line: Fast three hours prior to the start of a longer-duration event (60-90+ minutes). For shorter events, consuming a small amount of fuel an hour to two prior to the start may enhance performance.

SUMMARY

Though the recommendations outlined in this article may seem counterintuitive, they make perfect sense physiologically speaking. Apply them consistently and watch how well your body responds.

Over the years we've noted that most athletes are very skeptical about our pre-exercise recommendations, probably because it's a concept that they've never heard of before and/or because it doesn't appear to make sense. However, over the course of more than 24 years we can honestly say that we've yet to have one athlete tell us that the principles outlined in the article didn't work.

Applying these steps regarding pre-exercise calorie consumption for all your workouts will definitely enhance the quality of each and every one of them. Then, follow these same recommendations prior to your races and enjoy the distinct and noticeable advantage you'll have.

For more detailed and scientifically-referenced information regarding this topic, please read Dr. Misner's article "The Science Behind the Hammer Nutrition Pre-Race Meal Protocol," found in the Endurance Library portion of the KNOWLEDGE section at www.hammernutrition.com.

THE TOP 10

▶ The biggest mistakes
endurance athletes make

*Jeremy Milligan during the La Tierra
Torture in Santa Fe, New Mexico.
Photo : © James E. Rickman*

What am I doing wrong?

1. If you take all of the years of personal experience we've gained, the hundreds of research papers we've consulted, and the tens of thousands of endurance athletes we've coached, and then ignore every bit of that accumulated wisdom, you'll get the drift of this article.

2. **The mistakes that plague endurance athletes are all easily correctable with proper information and a little diligence in preparing your fueling strategy.**

3. Many, if not all, of these mistakes come from conventionally accepted practices and advice given by alleged "experts" in the field. **Our fueling philosophy often goes against the grain, but not against physiology or successful results.**

4. The ten biggest mistakes are:

Excess Hydration

Simple Sugar Consumption

Improper Amounts Of Calories

Inconsistent Electrolyte Supplementation

No Protein During Prolonged Exercise

Too Much Solid Food During Exercise

Using Something New In A Race Without Having Tested It In Training

Sticking With Your Game Plan When It's Not Working

Inadequate Post-Workout Nutrition

Improper Pre-Race Fueling

Start reading the full article on page 108

INTRODUCTION

There are obviously more than ten mistakes that an athlete can make—and in this latest incarnation of this article, you'll notice I've included an "honorable mention"—but those listed represent the most common performance-ruining gaffes.

As you read through each of these mistakes, at least some of them will sound painfully familiar. However, we don't just tell you what you're doing wrong; each of the ten topics also provides the appropriate corrective action. Follow this advice and you'll quickly see significant improvement in your overall performance.

FULL ARTICLE

Mistake #1:
Excess Hydration

Optimum nutritional support for endurance athletics means consuming the right amount of the right nutrients at the right time. You can neither overload nor undersupply your body without compromising athletic performance and incurring detrimental results. The principle of avoiding both too much and too little especially applies to hydration, where serious consequences occur from either mistake. If you don't drink enough, you'll suffer from unpleasant and performance-ruining dehydration. Drink too much, however, and you'll not only end up with impaired athletic performance, you may even be flirting with potentially life-threatening water intoxication.

One of the most respected researchers on hydration, Dr. Tim Noakes, studied the effects of thousands of endurance athletes and noted that the front-runners typically tend to dehydrate, while overhydration occurs most often among middle to back-of-the-pack athletes. Both conditions lead to hyponatremia (low blood sodium), but through different processes. Excess water consumption causes what is known as "dilutional hyponatremia," or an overly diluted level of sodium and electrolytes in the blood. This is as bad as under-hydrating in regards to increased potential for muscular cramping, but has the added disadvantages of stomach discomfort, bloating, and extra urine output. And, as mentioned earlier, in some unfortunate circumstances, excess hydration can lead to severe physiological circumstances, including death.

Unfortunately, endurance athletes too often adopt the "if a little is good, a lot is better" approach. This can lead to significant problems when you're trying to meet your hydration requirements. All it takes is one poor performance or DNF due to cramping and you start thinking,

"Hmm, maybe I didn't drink enough." Next thing you know, you're drinking so much water and fluids that your thirst is quenched but your belly is sloshing and you're still cramping. Remember, both undersupply and oversupply of fluid will get you in trouble.

How much should one drink? One expert, Dr. Ian Rogers, suggests that between 500-750 milliliters/hr (about 17-25 fluid ounces/hr) will fulfill most athletes'

hydration requirements under most conditions. I believe all athletes would benefit from what Dr. Rogers says: "Like most things in life, balance is the key and the balance is likely to be at a fluid intake not much above 500 milliliters (about 17 ounces) per hour in most situations, unless predicted losses are very substantial."

[Rogers, I.R. Fluid and Electrolyte Balance and Endurance Exercise: What can we learn from recent research? Wilderness Medicine Letter, 18:3, USA (2001)]

RECOMMENDATION

We at Hammer Nutrition have found that most athletes do very well under most conditions with a fluid intake of 20-25 ounces (approx 590-740 milliliters) per hour. Sometimes you may not need that much fluid—16-18 ounces (approx 473-532 ml) per hour may be quite acceptable. Sometimes you might need somewhat more, perhaps up to 28 ounces (approx 830 ml) hourly. Our position, however, is that the risk of dilutional hyponatremia increases substantially when an athlete repeatedly consumes more than 30 fluid ounces (nearly 890 ml) per hour. If more fluid intake is necessary (under very hot conditions, for example) proceed cautiously and remember to increase electrolyte intake as well to match your increased fluid intake. You can easily accomplish this by consuming a few additional Endurolytes capsules, or adding more scoops of Endurolytes Powder or Endurolytes Fizz tablets to your water/fuel bottle(s).

Photo : Kelly Pris

Mistake #2:
Simple Sugar Consumption

The Fast Lane

▶ Simple sugar-based drinks or gels have to be mixed and consumed at very dilute and calorically weak concentrations in order to be digested with any efficiency.

▶ Complex carbohydrates (polysaccharides) are the best choice for endurance athletes, as they allow your digestive system to rapidly and efficiently process a greater volume of calories, providing steady energy.

▶ Remove all processed simple sugar based fuels from your training and events. Processed simple sugars create havoc on the entire digestive system and body, which increases the stress placed on the body.

We believe that fructose, sucrose, glucose, and other simple sugars (mono- and disaccharides) are poor carbohydrate sources for fueling your body during exercise. Also, for optimal general health you should restrict your intake of these simple sugars (see the article "146 Reasons Sugar Ruins Your Health" in the Endurance Library portion of the KNOWLEDGE section at www.hammernutrition.com).

For endurance athletes, the primary problem with fuels containing simple sugars is that they must be mixed in weak 6-8% solutions in order to match body fluid osmolality parameters (280-303 mOsm) and thus be digested with any efficiency. Unfortunately, solutions mixed and consumed at this concentration only provide, at the most, about 100 calories per hour, inadequate for maintaining energy production on an hourly basis for most athletes. Using a 6-8% solution to obtain adequate calories means your fluid intake becomes so high that it causes discomfort and bloating, and you may possibly overhydrate to the point of fluid intoxication.

You can't make a "double or triple strength" mixture from a simple sugar-based carbohydrate fuel in the hopes of obtaining adequate calories because the concentration of that mixture, now far beyond the 6-8% mark, will remain in your stomach until sufficiently diluted, which may cause substantial stomach distress. You can drink more fluids in the hopes of "self diluting" the overly concentrated mixture, but remember that you'll increase the risk of overhydration. However, if you don't dilute with more water and electrolytes, your body will recruit these from other areas that critically need them and divert them to the digestive system to deal with the concentrated simple sugar mix. This can result in a variety of stomach-related distresses, not to mention increased cramping potential.

The bottom line is that simple sugar-based drinks or gels have to be mixed and consumed at very dilute and calorically weak concentrations in order to be digested with any efficiency. A simple sugar-based product used at a properly mixed concentration cannot provide adequate calories to sustain energy production. Any way you look at it, fuels containing simple sugars are inefficient and therefore not recommended during prolonged exercise.

Complex carbohydrates (polysaccharides) are the best choice for endurance athletes, as they allow your digestive system to rapidly and efficiently process a greater volume of calories, providing steady energy. Unlike simple sugars, which match body fluid osmolality at 6-8% solutions, complex carbohydrates match body fluid osmolality at substantially more concentrated 15-18% solutions. Even at this seemingly high concentration, complex carbohydrates (maltodextrins/glucose polymers) will empty the stomach at the same efficient rate as normal body fluids, providing up to three times more calories for energy production than simple sugar mixtures. This means that you can fulfill your caloric requirements without running the risk of overhydration or other stomach-related maladies.

RECOMMENDATION

To get the proper amount of easily digested calories, rely on fuels that use complex carbohydrates (maltodextrins or glucose polymers) only, with no added simple sugar as their carbohydrate source.

Hammer Gel and HEED are ideal for workouts and races up to two hours, sometimes longer under certain circumstances. For longer workouts and races, select Perpetuem or Sustained Energy as your primary fuel choice.

Mistake #3:
Improper Amounts Of Calories

▶ Your body can't replenish calories as fast as it expends them (ditto for fluids and electrolytes). Athletes who try to replace "calories out" with an equal amount of "calories in" usually suffer digestive maladies, with the inevitable poorer-than-expected outcome, and possibly the dreaded DNF ("Did Not Finish").

▶ During periods where fuel consumption may be less than your original hourly plan, body fat stores will effectively fill in the gap.

Too many endurance athletes fuel their bodies under the premise, "If I burn 500-800 calories an hour, I must consume that much or I'll bonk." However, repeating what Dr. Bill Misner stated earlier in *The GUIDE*, "To suggest that fluids, sodium, and fuels-induced glycogen replenishment can happen at the same rate as it is spent during exercise is simply not true. Endurance exercise beyond 1-2 hours is a deficit spending entity, with proportionate return or replenishment always in arrears. The endurance exercise outcome is to postpone fatigue, not to replace all the fuel, fluids, and electrolytes lost during the event. It can't be done, though many of us have tried." Simply put, your body can't replenish calories as fast as it expends them (ditto for fluids and electrolytes). Athletes who try to replace "calories out" with an equal or near equal amount of "calories in" usually suffer digestive maladies, with the inevitable poorer-than-expected outcome, and possibly the dreaded DNF ("Did Not Finish"). Body fat and glycogen stores easily fill the gap between energy output and fuel intake, so it's detrimental overkill to attempt calorie-for-calorie replacement.

Keep this in mind if you're doing ultra-endurance events, especially if you've had to "alter the game plan" and are unable to stick to your planned hourly caloric intake. For example, let's say you've been consuming an average of 250 calories an hour, but the heat or other circumstances (such as climbing a very long hill) prevent you from maintaining that desired hourly average. DO NOT try to "make up lost ground" by consuming additional calories; it's not only unnecessary, it may very well cause a lot of stomach distress, which will hurt your performance. Remember, during periods where fuel consumption may be less than your original hourly plan, body fat stores will effectively fill in the gap, thus eliminating the need to overcompensate with calories.

RECOMMENDATION

In general, an intake of 240-280 calories per hour is absolutely sufficient for the average size endurance athlete (approximately 160-165 lbs/approx 72.5-75 kg). Lighter weight athletes (<120-125 lbs/ approx 54.5-57 kg) will most certainly need less, while heavier athletes (>190 lbs/approx 86 kg) may need slightly more on occasion, the key word being "may."

When it comes to calorie intake, your focus should NOT be "How much can I consume before I get sick?" but rather, "What is the least amount of calories I need to keep my body doing what I want it to do hour after hour?" Start with our dosage recommendations as outlined in the article "*The Hammer Nutrition Fuels–What they are and how to use them*" (found in our supplementary booklet) and fine tune your intake as needed. As is the case in all aspects of fueling, when it comes to caloric intake you need to determine, via thorough testing under a variety of conditions, what amounts work best for you.

Amy Rappaport finishes the swim at the EagleMan Ironman 70.3 in Cambridge, Maryland.
Photo: ASI Photos

Mistake #4:

Inconsistent Electrolyte Supplementation

The Fast Lane

▶ Supplementing with only
one electrolyte or consuming
too much of one or more
electrolytic minerals
overrides the complex and
precise mechanisms that
regulate proper electrolyte
balance. The solution is
to provide the body with
a balanced blend of these
important minerals in a dose
that cooperates with and
enhances body mechanisms.

▶ Remember also that
electrolyte replenishment is
important even when it's not
hot outside.

Consuming sufficient amounts of calories and fluids during workouts and races is an obvious necessity. Consistent electrolyte supplementation is equally important. Just as your car's engine requires sufficient oil to keep its many parts running smoothly, your body requires electrolytic minerals to maintain smooth performance of vital functions such as muscle contraction. Athletes who neglect this important component of fueling will impair their performance, and may incur painful and debilitating cramping and spasms, a sure way to ruin a workout or race.

However, this doesn't mean that athletes should indiscriminately ingest copious amounts of one or more electrolytes; sodium (salt) is usually the most misused. Supplementing with only one electrolyte or consuming too much of one or more electrolytic minerals overrides the complex and precise mechanisms that regulate proper electrolyte balance. The solution is to provide the body with a balanced blend of these important minerals in a dose that cooperates with and enhances body mechanisms. Salt tablets alone cannot sufficiently satisfy electrolyte requirements, and excess salt consumption will cause more problems than it resolves.

Additionally, remeber that electrolyte replenishment is important even when it's not hot outside. Sure, you may not need as much as you would in hotter weather, but your body still requires consistent replenishment of these minerals to maintain the optimal performance of many important bodily functions. You don't wait until you dehydrate before you drink fluids, or until you bonk before you put some calories back in your body, do you? Of course not. You fulfill your fueling requirements before the consequences of inadequate replenishment strike. The same principle applies to electrolyte replenishment. Going back to the engine/oil analogy, you don't wait until the engine seizes before refilling the oil reservoir. The same is true for electrolytes, the body's "motor oil," in that you don't want to wait until you start cramping before you replenish these important minerals.

RECOMMENDATION

Endurolytes, in capsule, effervescent tablet, or powder form, is an inexpensive, easy-to-dose, and easy-to-consume way to get your necessary electrolytes. Use Endurolytes consistently during workouts and races to fulfill this crucial fueling need.

Matt Butterfield, of the Hammer Nutrition Factory Racing Team, rides the course prior to the 24 Hours of Moab. Photo : Brad Lamson

The Fast Lane

▶ While carbohydrates are still the primary component of your fuel, it should include a small amount of protein when training sessions or races last longer than two to three hours.

Mistake #5:
No Protein During Prolonged Exercise

When exercise extends beyond about two hours, your body begins to utilize some protein to fulfill its energy requirements, as you begin to derive glucose from amino acids. This metabolic process helps to satisfy anywhere from 5-15% of your energy needs. If you fail to include protein in your fuel, your body has only one other choice: your own muscle! Called "lean muscle tissue catabolism" or "muscle cannibalization," this process devastates performance through muscle deterioration and increased fatigue-causing ammonia accumulation, and also negatively affects the immune system and recovery. The longer your workout or race, the greater these problems are compounded. While carbohydrates are still the primary

Thoughts on protein intake

"Soy's remarkable donation to endurance performance is deserving of our review. Soy has been observed to produce a higher degree of uric acid content than whey proteins. Uric acid is reduced by excessive free radicals produced during exercise. When uric acid levels are higher, that is an indication of less free radical release due to antioxidant influence of the isoflavones found exclusively in soy. This is one reason why soy may be the preferred dietary protein application during endurance exercise."

- William Misner, Ph.D. - Director of Research & Product Development, Emeritus

Article continues here

component of your fuel, it should include a small amount of protein when training sessions or races last longer than two to three hours.

We believe that soy protein's amino acid profile is ideal for use during exercise, which is why Hammer Nutrition's Perpetuem and Sustained Energy contain soy as the protein source. For instance, compared to whey protein (which is ideal for recovery), soy protein has higher levels of phenylalanine and tyrosine, which may aid in maintaining alertness during ultra-distance races. Soy protein has higher amounts of histidine, which is part of the beta-alanyl l-histidine dipeptide known as carnosine, which has antioxidant/acid buffering benefits. Finally, soy protein has higher levels of aspartic acid, which plays an important role in energy production via the Krebs cycle.

RECOMMENDATION

Using Perpetuem or Sustained Energy as your primary fuel during workouts and races longer than two to three hours will satisfy energy requirements from a precise ratio of complex carbohydrates and soy protein, the latter of which helps protect against excess muscle breakdown. You stay healthier, reduce soreness, and decrease recovery time.

> Exercise diminishes
> digestive system function,
> so regular solid food intake
> should be limited in your
> fueling strategy.

Mistake #6:
Too Much Solid Food During Exercise

In the 1985 Race Across America (RAAM), Jonathan Boyer rode to victory using a liquid diet as his primary fuel source. Since then, it has become the norm for endurance and ultra-endurance athletes. Liquid nutrition is the easiest, most convenient, and most easily digested way to get a calorie and nutrient-dense fuel. Solid food, for the most part, cannot match the precision or nutrient density of the best liquid fuels. In addition, too much solid food consumption will divert blood from working muscles for the digestive process. This, along with the amount of digestive enzymes, fluids, and time required in breaking down the constituents of solid food, can cause bloating, nausea, and/or lethargy. Lastly, some of the calories ingested from solid foods are used up simply to break down

Pay Attention!

If you choose to consume solid food during your workouts or races, even during ultra-distance events, we suggest you heed these two recommendations:

1. Choose foods that have little or no refined sugar or saturated fats. Don't think, "I'm a calorie burning machine so I can eat anything I want . . . calories are calories." Remember, what you put in your body greatly determines what you get out of it. The well-known phrase "garbage in, garbage out" fully applies here.

2. Use solid food sparingly, and only as an exception or diversion. Maintain your primary intake through liquid/gel sources.

• •

Article continues here

and digest them; in essence, these calories are wasted.

Occasional solid food intake provides a welcome diversion during ultra-endurance efforts, but we don't recommend it as your primary fuel source. In fact, our position is that NO solid food is necessary (even food as healthy as the Hammer Bar) during workouts or races in the 12-hour-or-under range.

RECOMMENDATION

Use Hammer Gel, HEED, Sustained Energy, and/or Perpetuem as your primary fuel source during exercise. These provide precise amounts of specific nutrients and are designed for easy digestion, rapid nutrient utilization, and less chance of stomach distress. Also, the numerous flavors and mixing options give you plenty of variety. If you do decide to consume solid food, use it sparingly and select high-quality foods such as the Hammer Bar.

Mistake #7:

Using Something New In A Race Without Having Tested It In Training

The Fast Lane

▶ Unless you're absolutely desperate and willing to accept the consequences, do not try anything new in competition.

▶ Use Hammer Nutrition fuels, try all sorts of combinations in training, and keep a log of what works best for you.

The title is pretty self-explanatory; it's one of THE cardinal rules for all athletes, yet you'd be amazed at how many break it. Are you guilty as well? Unless you're absolutely desperate and willing to accept the consequences, do not try anything new in competition, be it equipment, fuel, or tactics. These all must be tested and refined in training.

RECOMMENDATION

Because all of the Hammer Nutrition fuels are complementary (they all work well alone or in combination), you have all the flexibility you need to ensure that you can tailor a fueling program for any length of race, regardless of the conditions. You'll never have to guess or grab something off the aid station table in the hopes of trying to keep going for another hour. Use Hammer Nutrition fuels, try a variety of combinations in training, and keep a log of what works best for you. If you expand your training log to include fuel intake also, you'll have the data you need to prepare a smart fueling protocol for your next event.

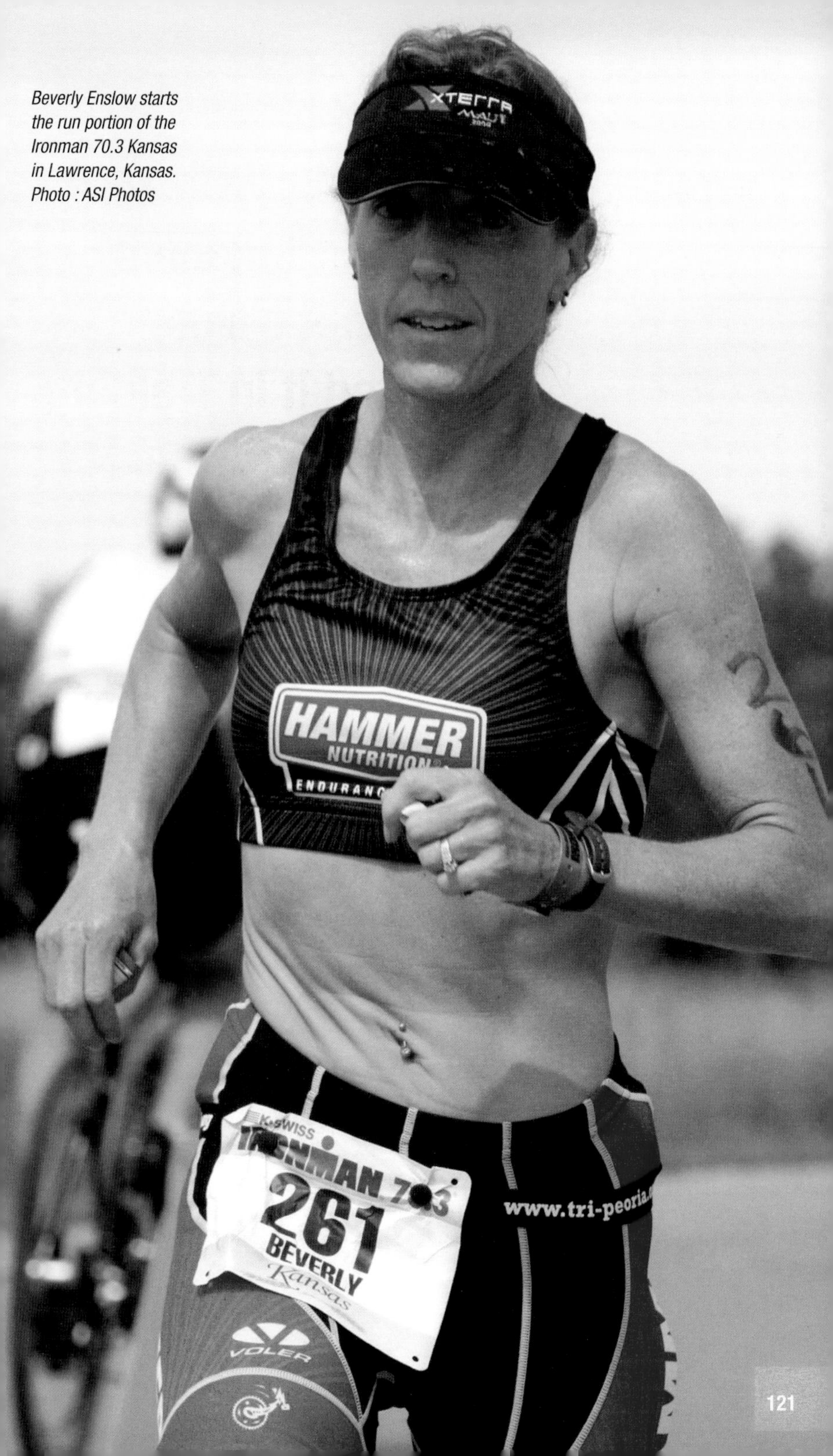

Beverly Enslow starts the run portion of the Ironman 70.3 Kansas in Lawrence, Kansas. Photo : ASI Photos

▶ During the heat, it becomes more important to stay hydrated and maintain adequate electrolyte levels, so be willing to cut back on calorie consumption.

▶ What does fine in terms of fueling—your hourly intake of fluids, calories, and electrolytes—during training at a slower pace and lower overall energy output, might fail during competition.

▶ Many athletes think that the cure for a poor race is to train harder and longer. A better tactic is to recuperate completely after your race, evaluating what went right and what went wrong during the race, and adapting your training accordingly.

Mistake #8:

Sticking With Your Game Plan Even When It's Not Working

Endurance athletes tend to be strong-willed and uncompromising. Most strive to have a "game plan" in place for their training program, which is, of course, an excellent idea. Smart athletes also have a strategy for their supplements and fueling. Having this nutritional game plan that you've honed during training is a big step toward success on race day, but don't slavishly adhere to it during the race if it's not working. What does fine in terms of fueling—your hourly intake of fluids, calories, and electrolytes—during training at a slower pace and lower overall energy output, might fail during competition. Athletes who stubbornly maintain the same fuel intake hour after hour, even when it's clearly not working, end up with poorer results, if they finish at all.

Yes, it's important to maintain consistent caloric intake during a workout or race, but if the weather gets hot, the body's ability to process calories usually diminishes. It's important to recognize this and to listen to your body. Continuing to force down "X" amount of calories an hour (the original "game plan"), especially under extreme conditions when your body cannot properly assimilate them, puts a burden on your stomach and can cause any number of stomach-related maladies, which will certainly hinder or ruin performance. In the heat, it becomes more important to stay hydrated and maintain adequate electrolyte levels, so be willing to cut back on calorie consumption. Body fat stores, which satisfy up to two-thirds of energy requirements during prolonged exercise, will accommodate energy needs during occasional breaks from regular intervals of fuel consumption. During the heat, fueling is still important, but the focus shifts towards maintaining hydration and proper electrolyte levels. Resume regular caloric intake when you start feeling more acclimated to the heat and your stomach has had some time to assimilate the fuel that it already has.

In a similar, but non-fueling vein, another time when it's not a wise idea to stick to your training plan is after you've had a poorer-than-expected race. Many athletes think that the cure for a poor race is to train harder and longer. Instead of recuperating, many athletes will train themselves into the ground, usually ending up not fitter, but overtrained, with a poorly functioning immune system. A better tactic is to recuperate completely after your race, evaluating what went right and what went wrong during the race, then adapting your training accordingly; training harder and longer isn't necessarily your best option. Remember that recovery is as important a part of your training and the achievement of your athletic goals as the actual training session. Make sure that you take your recovery as seriously as your training.

RECOMMENDATION

It's a good practice to have a game plan that includes a fueling protocol that you have refined during training, but you need to be flexible. Evaluate and adjust accordingly as race pace and weather dictate. Have a game plan, but "write it in pencil, not in ink."

Ultra athlete, Suzy Degazon, competes in her 13th consecutive Ultraman Triathlon on the Big Island of Hawaii. Photo : Timothy Carlson

Mistake #9:
Inadequate Post-Workout Nutrition

The Fast Lane

▶ Carbohydrate replenishment as soon as possible upon completion of a workout takes advantage of high glycogen synthase activity, imperative to maximizing muscle glycogen, the first fuel the body uses when exercise commences.

▶ Protein supplies the amino acids necessary to:

- maximize glycogen storage potential

- rebuild and repair muscle tissue

- support optimal immune system function

Performance improvement depends on a program of exercise that stimulates muscular and cardiovascular adaptation followed by a recovery period in which the body rebuilds itself slightly more fit than before. Thus, the real gain of exercise occurs during recovery, but only in the presence of adequate rest and nutritional support. Athletes who fail to replenish carbohydrates and protein shortly after workouts will never obtain full value from their efforts. So even though all you may want to do after a hard workout is get horizontal and not move for several hours, you must first take care of what might be the most important part of your workout: the replenishment of carbohydrates and protein.

Carbohydrate replenishment as soon as possible upon completion of a workout (ideally within the first 30-60 minutes) takes advantage of high glycogen synthase activity, imperative to maximizing muscle glycogen, the first fuel the body uses when exercise commences. Protein supplies the amino acids necessary to (a) maximize glycogen storage potential, (b) rebuild and repair muscle tissue, and (c) support optimal immune system function.

This is also an ideal time to provide the body with cellular protection support in the form of antioxidants. Because athletes use several times more oxygen than sedentary people, they are more prone to oxidative damage, which not only impairs recovery but is also considered a main cause of degenerative diseases. Consistent supplementation with a full spectrum vitamin/mineral supplement, along with any additional antioxidants, boosts

✱ Article Reference
"RECOVERY–A crucial component for athletic success."
Page 74

and maintains the immune system and reduces recovery time.

The bottom line is that post-workout nutrition is an important component of your routine, and properly done, allows you to obtain maximum benefit from your training. For more detailed information on this extremely important topic, please refer to the article "RECOVERY–A crucial component for athletic success."*

RECOMMENDATION

Depending on a number of factors (such as body size and length/intensity of the workout), consume 30-90 grams of complex carbohydrates and 10-30 grams of protein (a 3:1 ratio of carbohydrates to protein) immediately after workouts. This is easily accomplished with Recoverite, the all-in-one, complex carbohydrate/glutamine-fortified whey protein isolate recovery drink. Supplements to consider for providing antioxidants and supporting enhanced recovery are the Hammer Nutrition products Premium Insurance Caps, Race Caps Supreme, Mito Caps, Super Antioxidant, AO Booster, and Xobaline.

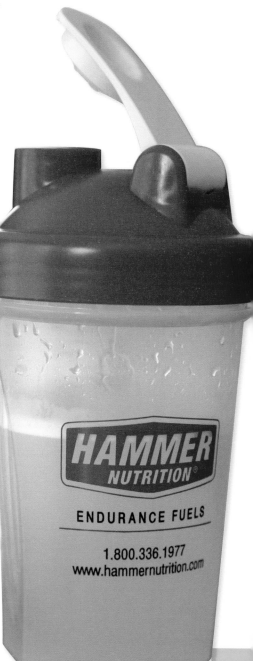

HAMMER NUTRITION®

ENDURANCE FUELS

1.800.336.1977
www.hammernutrition.com

Improper Pre-Workout/Race Fueling

Far too often, athletes put themselves at a "metabolic disadvantage" during a workout or race by fueling improperly prior to it. The article "PROPER FUELING–Pre-workout & race suggestions"* discusses this in greater detail, but we mention it here as well because it's definitely one of the biggest fueling errors that athletes make. It's also one that is easy to remedy. Let's look at the three primary factors:

1. **Overconsuming food the night before a race or workout in the hopes of "carbo loading"** – It would be nice if you could maximize muscle glycogen stores the night before a race or tough workout; unfortunately, human physiology doesn't work that way. Increasing and maximizing muscle glycogen stores takes many weeks of consistent training and post-workout fuel replenishment. Carbohydrates consumed in excess the night before will only be eliminated or stored as body fat (dead weight).

2. **Overconsuming calories in your pre-workout/race meal** – The goal of pre-exercise calorie consumption is to top off your liver glycogen, which has been depleted during your sleep. Believe it or not, to accomplish this you don't need to eat a mega-calorie meal (600, 800, 1000 calories or more), as some would have you believe. A preworkout/race meal of 200-400 calories–comprised of complex carbohydrates, perhaps a small amount

* Article Reference
"PROPER FUELING– Pre-workout & race suggestions"
Page 96

of soy or rice protein, little or no fiber or fat, and consumed three or more hours prior to the start—is quite sufficient. You can't add anything to muscle glycogen stores at this time so stuffing yourself is counterproductive, especially if you've got an early morning workout or race start.

3. **Eating a pre-race meal at the wrong time** – Let's assume that you've been really good – you've been training hard, yet wisely, and replenishing your body with adequate amounts of high-quality calories as soon as possible after every workout. As a result, you've now built up a nice 60-90 minute reservoir of muscle glycogen, the first fuel your body will use when the race begins. A sure way to deplete those hard-earned glycogen stores too rapidly is to eat a meal (or an energy bar, gel, or sports drink) an hour or two prior to the start of the race.

RECOMMENDATION

Don't go overboard with your food consumption the night before a workout or race. Especially important for races is the adherence to these two rules:

1. Eat clean, which means no refined sugar (skip dessert or eat fruit), low or no saturated fats, and no alcohol.
2. Eat until you're satisfied, but not more.

If you're going to have a meal the morning of your workout or race, you need to eat an appropriate amount of calories (don't overdo it), and finish all calorie consumption at least three hours prior to the start of the workout or race. If that's not logistically feasible, have a small amount (100-200 calories) of easily digested complex carbohydrates 5-10 minutes prior to the start. Either of these strategies will help top off liver glycogen stores (which again, is the goal of pre-exercise calorie consumption) without negatively affecting how your body burns its muscle glycogen.

The Fast Lane

▶ Don't drink excessive amounts of water in the hopes of getting a head start on your fluid requirements for a race.

Don't stuff yourself with extra food in the hopes of "carbo loading."

Don't consume extra sodium in the hopes of "topping off your body stores" prior to a race.

▶ Avoid the temptation to train too much and/or too close to race day. You will not be able to positively influence your fitness level in the days leading up to the race; however, you can negatively impact your race by training during that time.

Honorable Mention:
Overcompensating In The Days Leading Up To A Race

Far too many athletes overdo it in terms of calorie, fluid, and salt consumption in the days leading up to a race, thinking they're getting a head start on their fueling needs come race day. Big mistake! Here are the fueling/diet-specific areas to focus on and our recommendations on how to avoid these commonly-made mistakes:

• **FLUIDS** – Don't drink excessive amounts of water in the hopes of having them available for a race. Consumption of roughly 0.5 to 0.6 of your body weight is a good gauge of how much water you should be consuming daily (Example: A 180 lb/approx 82 kg athlete should drink roughly 90-108 ounces of water daily.) However, if you haven't been following this recommendation consistently, don't start now, as this will overwhelm your body with too much fluid too soon, which may increase the potential for hyponatremia.

• **CALORIES** – As discussed in #10, don't stuff yourself with extra food in the hopes of "carbo loading." The time period for carbohydrate loading (i.e., maximizing muscle glycogen storage capabilities) has, for all intents and purposes, passed. In essence, "carbo loading" is what you did in the 0-60 minutes after all of your training sessions. That's when the glycogen synthase enzyme—which controls glycogen storage—is most active, and that's how you topped off your glycogen stores. Any excess food that you eat in the days leading up to a race is either going to be passed through the bowels or stored in adipose cells . . . neither of those things will benefit you.

- **SODIUM** – Don't consume extra sodium (salt) in the hopes of "topping off your body stores" prior to a race. Since the average American already consumes approximately 6,000-8,000 mg per day (if not more), an amount well above the maximum recommended dose of 2,300-2,400 mg per day, there is absolutely no need to increase that amount in the days prior to a race. (Hint: Adopting a low-sodium diet will do wonders for both your health and athletic performance.) High sodium intake is a recipe for disaster because it will greatly increase the potential for disruption of the hormonal mechanisms that control sodium regulation, recirculation, and conservation. Be especially cognizant of the salt content in your foods, especially if you go out to eat. Dining out can easily increase your already-high salt intake dramatically (into double figures!).

On a non-diet/fueling note, avoid the temptation to train too much and/or too close to race day. You will not be able to positively influence your fitness level in the days leading up to a race; however, you can negatively impact your race by training during this time (training meaning anything of significant duration or intensity). As well-known coach Jeff Cuddeback states, "If you think you're going to further your fitness through training the week of your key race, you're sadly mistaken. If you are the type to train right up to the event, you will almost certainly underperform."

The best performances in long-duration events are achieved by getting to the starting line well rested rather than "razor sharp." In doing so, you may find yourself not hitting on all cylinders during those first few minutes. In fact, you might even struggle a bit. However, your body will not forget all of the training you've done and it will absolutely reward you for giving it the time it needed to "soak up" all of that training.

Laura Labelle enters the pool in preparation for a race. Photo : Brian Wadley

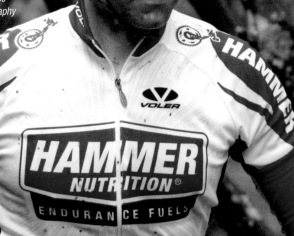

PROTEIN

Why it's important for endurance athletes

Jamie Ingalls carries his bike through a section of the Cohutta 100 in Ducktown, Tennessee
Photo : Blue Basin Photography

Pay attention to protein

1. Endurance athletes often focus on carbohydrate intake, and leave protein considerations for the weight lifters and bodybuilders. Differences in goals and body type aside, the fact is that **endurance athletes also need a considerable amount of protein.**

2. **Endurance exercise creates two protein demands.** One is to repair and rebuild muscle tissue; the other is to protect and enhance immune system functioning.

3. **Lean muscle mass can be lost at a considerable rate during exercise, especially if protein is deficient in the fueling.**

4. Lengthy training sessions greatly stress the immune system. **Athletes with inadequate protein intake are susceptible to overtraining syndrome, overuse injuries, slow healing of injuries, and catching colds and other ailments.**

5. **Whey protein, because of its fast absorption, is the ideal recovery protein for post-exercise use. Soy is best during exercise**, as it contains high amounts of "beneficial during exercise" amino acids. Additionally, unlike glutamine-fortified whey protein, soy is less likely to produce ammonia, which in turn contributes to muscle fatigue.

6. To determine your optimal protein intake (in grams), multiply your body weight in kilograms (pounds divided by 2.2) by 1.4 to 1.7, depending on the intensity of your exercise.

Start reading the full article on page 132

INTRODUCTION

Are you an endurance athlete who believes that protein supplementation is strictly for weight lifters, bodybuilders, and purely-strength athletes? If so, it's vitally important to understand that hard-training endurance athletes also need a substantial amount of protein in their daily diets. This article focuses on how to obtain adequate amounts of the proper protein at the right time to satisfy the specific needs of endurance athletes.

FULL ARTICLE

Endurance athletes need more than just carbohydrates

Endurance athletes tend to focus on carbohydrate intake and pay little, if any, attention to protein. As a result, protein deficiency appears often among endurance athletes, with its inevitable negative effects on performance and health. Serious endurance athletes do need considerable amounts of protein, far above the normal adult RDA, because maintenance, repair, and growth of lean muscle mass all depend on it, as well as optimum immune system function. Low dietary protein lengthens recovery time, causes muscle weakness, and suppresses the immune system. Chronic protein deficiency will cancel the beneficial effects of your workouts; instead, you will become susceptible to fatigue, lethargy, anemia, and possibly even more severe disorders. Athletes with over training syndrome usually have protein deficiency.

Protein use during exercise

As discussed in the article "CALORIC INTAKE–Proper amounts during endurance exercise" on page 54, it's important that the workout fuel contains a small amount of protein when exercise gets into the second hour and beyond. Research [Lemon, PWR "Protein and Exercise Update" 1987, Medicine and Science in Sports and Exercise. 1987;19 (Suppl): S 179-S 190.] has shown that exercise burns up to 15% of the total amount of calories from protein by extracting particular amino acids from muscle tissues. If the endurance athlete does not provide this protein as part of the fuel mixture, more lean muscle tissue will be sacrificed through gluconeogenesis to provide fuel and preserve biochemical balance. Simply put, when you exercise beyond 2-3 hours, you need to provide protein from a dietary source or your body will "borrow" amino acids from your muscle tissue. The longer you exercise, the more muscle tissue is sacrificed. This creates performance problems both during exercise (due to increased levels of fatigue-causing ammonia) and during your post-exercise recovery (due to excess lean muscle tissue damage).

Bottom line: During exercise

Article continues on page 134

Protein
Questions, concerns, & answers

In addition to the usual information we offer concerning all of our fuels and supplements, the issue of protein intake also requires dealing with some misperceptions. Endurance athletes have certain oft-spoken beliefs about protein intake; here we take a look at the three most commonly voiced.

"I thought only bodybuilders needed high protein diets."

When you get down to it, however, we are bodybuilders in some respects, building our bodies to do what we want them to. The truth is that endurance athletes and bodybuilders have similar protein requirements, but the way in which the body uses the protein differs. Bodybuilders need protein primarily to increase muscle tissue; endurance athletes need protein primarily to repair existing muscle tissue that is undergoing constant breakdown from day-to-day training.

"Eating a high-protein diet will cause unwanted weight gain and muscle growth."

Actually, the type of training you engage in determines whether you bulk up or not. High volume endurance training does not produce muscle bulk, regardless of protein intake, whereas relatively low volumes of strength training will. Either way, the muscle tissue requires protein. Additionally, it is the volume of calories you consume—be it from carbohydrates, protein, or fat—that is the primary factor in weight gain. You've simply got to have more calories going out (i.e. "being burned") during exercise and other activities than you have coming in via the diet to avoid unwanted weight gain.

"But I thought carbohydrates were the most important fuel for exercise."

While carbohydrates are indeed the body's preferred source of fuel, protein plays an important part in the energy and muscle preservation needs of endurance athletes. Protein is mainly known for its role in the repair, maintenance, and growth of body tissues, but it also has a role in energy supply. After about 90 minutes of exercise in well-trained athletes, muscle glycogen stores become nearly depleted, and the body will look for alternative fuel sources. Your own muscle tissue becomes a target for a process called gluconeogenesis, which is the synthesis of glucose from the fatty and amino acids of lean muscle tissue. The degree of soreness and stiffness after a long, intense workout is a good indicator of just how much muscle cannibalization you have incurred. Adding protein to your fuel mix provides amino acids and thus reduces tissue cannibalization.

Article continues here

The Fast Lane

....

▶ Whey protein is the premier protein for recovery and enhanced immune system function.

Soy protein is ideal for fulfilling protein requirements prior to and during endurance exercise.

....

▶ BCAAs and glutamic acid, both found in significant quantity in soy protein, aid in the replenishing of glutamine within the body, and without the risk of ammonia production caused by orally ingested glutamine, an amino acid usually added to whey protein.

....

that extends beyond two hours, the wise endurance athlete will make sure that complex carbohydrate and protein intake are both adequate to delay and offset this cannibalization process.

What kind to use?

Which protein is best for use before, during, and after exercise has been a subject of much debate. We recommend a combination of both soy and whey protein, used at separate times, to provide the most comprehensive support for an endurance athlete's diet. We believe that whey protein is the premier protein for recovery and enhanced immune system function, while soy protein is ideal for fulfilling protein requirements prior to and during endurance exercise. This doesn't mean that using soy protein for recovery purposes would be "wrong" or in any way harmful. For optimal benefits, though, you won't find a better protein for recovery and immune system boosting than whey protein, in particular whey protein isolate. For exercise-specific benefits it's hard to top soy, which is the main reason we use it in both Sustained Energy and Perpetuem.

The benefits of soy protein

Because it has less potential than whey protein to produce ammonia, a primary cause of muscle fatigue, soy protein is best used prior to and during exercise. This alone would make soy the preferential choice for use during exercise, but soy has yet more benefits.

As mentioned in the "CALORIC INTAKE– Proper amounts during endurance exercise"* article, soy protein has a unique amino acid profile. This composition adds to its attractiveness as the ideal protein to use during endurance exercise. Although not as high in concentration as whey protein, soy

* Article Reference
"CALORIC INTAKE–
Proper amounts during
endurance exercise"
Page 54

Soy Protein vs. Whey Protein

A comparison (approximate amounts per gram of protein) of "during exercise"-specific amino acids

Amino Acid	Soy Protein	Whey Protein
Glutamic Acid	138 mg	103 mg
Alanine	31 mg	9 mg
Histidine	19 mg	16 mg
Aspartic Acid	84 mg	78 mg
Phenylalnine	38 mg	32 mg
Tyrosine	27 mg	7 mg

Article continues here

protein still provides a substantial amount of branched chain amino acids (BCAAs), which your body readily converts for energy production. BCAAs and glutamic acid, another amino acid found in significant quantity in soy protein, also help replenish glutamine in the body, without the risk of ammonia production caused by orally ingested glutamine, an amino acid usually added to whey protein. Soy has high amounts of both alanine and histidine, which is part of the beta-alanyl l-histidine dipeptide known as carnosine, renowned for its antioxidant and acid buffering benefits. Soy protein also has a high level of aspartic acid, which plays an important role in energy production via the Krebs cycle. Lastly, soy protein has higher levels of phenylalanine and tyrosine than does whey, which may aid in maintaining alertness during extreme ultra distance races. See Table A above.

Willie Zellmer of Team Hammer/CMG.
Photo : Angela Miller

▶ Comparing cancer rates for the U.S. to those of Asian countries which have soy-rich diets:

- Japan has 1/4 the rate of breast cancer and 1/5 the rate of prostate cancer

- Medical researches in China linked the consumption of soy milk to a 50% risk reduction for stomach cancer

- Studies done in Hong Kong suggest that daily soy consumption was a primary factor in a 50% reduction in the incidence of lung cancer

In addition, for general health benefits it's hard to beat soy. Soy protein contains multitudes of health-enhancing phytochemicals. Scientific research has established many connections between soy consumption and lower rates of certain cancers, notably breast, prostate, stomach, lung, and colon. Comparing cancer rates for the U.S. to those of Asian countries (which have soy-rich diets) shows some remarkable differences. For instance, Japan has one-fourth the rate of breast cancer and one-fifth the rate of prostate cancer. In China, medical researchers linked the consumption of soy milk to a 50% risk reduction for stomach cancer. Studies done in Hong Kong suggest that daily soy consumption was a primary factor in a 50% reduction in the incidence of lung cancer.

Soy Protein - Friend or Foe?

Even though the just-mentioned benefits attributed to soy protein are generally accepted by the majority, there is an ongoing debate as to whether or not soy protein is truly beneficial. Some tout soy as being a super-healthy protein source, while others decry it as being responsible for a variety of undesirable effects. Perhaps the most highly debated topic is in regards to soy's naturally occurring phytoestrogens and whether or not they negatively affect hormone levels (particularly in males), causing an imbalance leading to increased estrogen levels. Dr. Bill Misner comments, noting that there are those who do not agree with his position:

> Phytoestrogens from plant lignans or isoflavonoids from at least 15 plants behave within the body like weak estrogens. Phytoestrogens are so chemically similar to estrogen that they bind to the estrogen receptors on the cells within the body. It should be emphasized that they do not initiate the same biological effects that true estrogens exert.

Phytoestrogens paradoxically act as antiestrogens, effectively diluting the impact of the body's own production of estrogen, because they occupy the same receptor sites (estradiol receptor sites) that would otherwise be occupied by endogenous estrogen. Therefore, plant phytoestrogens protect the body from the detrimental effects of excessive estrogen. The healthy foods and supplements that introduce phytoestrogens into the diet are Mexican wild yam, black cohosh, red clover, licorice, sage, unicorn root, soy, flax seeds, and even tiny sesame seeds. None of these foods are associated with behavioral change or hormonal modification.

Consuming GMO-free soy protein generates anabolic sequences desirable for the health-conscious male and female endurance athlete, especially those over age 40. If allergenic, thyroid, or digestion issues are present, then another protein should be selected. Soy's phytoestrogen properties block the effects of potent endogenous estrogens, with no known gender effects to males or females as reported from the literature. The net result from soy protein consumption is anabolic lean muscle mass gain. While I regard soy as an excellent dietary protein, alternating soy with other lean dietary proteins during training presents a responsible and defendable rationale.

Each scoop of Hammer Soy provides 25 grams of the highest quality, 100% GMO (genetically modified organism)-free soy protein, without any fillers, added sugar, or artificial sweeteners or flavoring. Hammer Soy's highly concentrated nature makes it a hunger-satisfying addition anytime, helping you to easily fulfill your daily protein requirements. Add Hammer Soy to juices, smoothies, or other soy-based drinks to make a satisfying and healthy meal. It's also a great

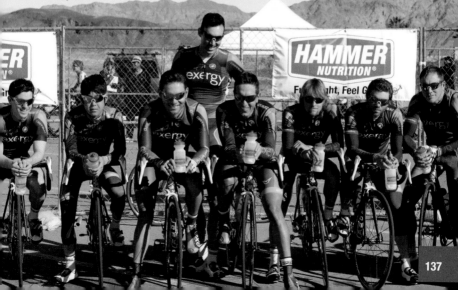

Team Exergy shows what fuels them at the Calville Bay Classic.
Photo : Kristy Bako

Whey Protein vs. Soy Protein

A comparison (approximate amounts per gram of protein) of "after exercise"-specific amino acids

Amino Acid	Whey Protein	Soy Protein
Leucine	100 mg	56 mg
Isoleucine	51 mg	35 mg
Valine	36 mg	16 mg
Methionine	17 mg	9 mg
Cysteine	33 mg	9 mg

The Fast Lane

▶ Whey protein concentrate contains anywhere from 70% to 80% actual protein (and, sadly, sometimes even less), the remainder being fat and lactose. Isolate, on the other hand, contains 90% - 97+% protein—with little, if any, lactose or fat—making it the purest form of whey protein available.

* Article Reference "RECOVERY–A crucial component for success" Page 74

Article continues here

addition when making pancake or muffin batter, adding high-quality, all-vegetable protein to the mixture.

The benefits of whey protein

For enhancing the recovery process, whey protein has no peer. As mentioned in the article, "RECOVERY–A crucial component for success,"* whey protein has the highest biological value (BV) of any protein source. BV rates the availability of the protein once ingested, and whey is arguably the most rapidly absorbed protein, exactly what you want post-workout. Whey protein's amino acid profile contains the highest percentage of essential amino acids, 25% of which are the BCAAs leucine, isoleucine, and valine, the most important for muscle tissue repair. Whey is also a rich source of two other important amino acids, methionine and cysteine, which stimulate the natural production of glutathione, one of the body's most powerful antioxidants and a major player in maintaining a strong immune system. Glutathione also supports healthy liver function. See Table B above.

Article continues on page 140

Hammer protein tips

Recovery/Meal Replacement Formulas

1 rounded scoop of Hammer Whey (equal to about 1.25 scoops) with 3 servings (approx. 5 tablespoons) of Hammer Gel in 8-10 ounces of water. This provides approximately 370 calories from approximately 22.5 grams of protein and approximately 66 grams of carbohydrates.

3-4 scoops of Sustained Energy with 1/2 scoop of Hammer Whey in 16 ounces of water. This provides roughly 360-467 calories from approximately 19-23 grams of protein and 68-91 grams of carbohydrates.

2-3 scoops of Sustained Energy with 1 scoop of Hammer Whey in 8 ounces of organic orange juice. This provides approximately 413-520 calories from approximately 27-30 grams of protein and approximately 71-94 grams of carbs.

Pre-workout/race meals

1/2 scoop of Hammer Soy with 2-3 servings (approximately 3.5-5 tablespoons) of Hammer Gel in water. This yields approximately 44-66 grams of carbohydrates and approximately 12.5 grams of protein equaling roughly 235-325 calories.

1/3 scoop of Hammer Soy with 2-2.5 scoops of Sustained Energy in water. This yields approximately 45-57 grams of carbohydrates and approximately 15-16.5 grams of protein equaling roughly 250-304 calories.

3 scoops of Sustained Energy in water supplies 320 calories from 68 grams of carbohydrates and 10 grams of protein.

2-2.5 scoops of Perpetuem in water provides 270-337.5 calories from 54-67.5 grams of carbohydrates and 7-8.75 grams of protein. Note: Before cold weather workouts or races, a WARM bottle of Caffè Latte Perpetuem is the ticket!

The Fast Lane

▶ To find out how much protein you require, multiply your weight in kilograms by 1.4 to 1.7, depending on your exercise intensity. This gives you the amount of protein (in grams) that you should consume on a daily basis. (To convert from pounds to kilograms, divide by 2.2.)

▶ Track and record your diet and do some calculating. It takes quite a bit of effort to ensure adequate protein intake, especially for vegetarians and those who avoid dairy products.

▶ If you're serious about your performance and also your health, then respect the importance of providing adequate protein in your diet.

Article continues here

Hammer Whey

Each scoop of Hammer Whey contains 18 grams of 100% micro-filtered whey protein isolate, with no added fillers, sugar, or artificial sweeteners or flavoring. The key word here is isolate. Manufacturers supply two forms of whey–isolate and concentrate. Whey protein concentrate contains anywhere from 70% to 80% actual protein (and, sadly, sometimes even less), the remainder being fat and lactose. Isolate, on the other hand, contains 90%-97+% protein–with little, if any, lactose or fat–making it the purest form of whey protein available. Because isolate contains almost no lactose, even those with lactose intolerance find it an easily digestible protein source. We use only isolate in our whey-containing products, Hammer Whey and Recoverite.

In addition, each scoop of Hammer Whey contains a whopping six grams of glutamine, a remarkable amino acid. Space limits all that could be written regarding the benefits of this extraordinary, multi-beneficial amino acid, but needless to say, it's essential for endurance athletes in supporting enhanced recovery and immune system function. Glutamine is the most abundant amino acid in your muscles. Intense exercise severely depletes glutamine, which makes supplementation so important. Glutamine plays a significant role in the glycogen synthesis process, and along with the branched chain amino acids, glutamine helps repair and rebuild muscle tissue. In addition, glutamine has been shown to help raise endogenous levels of glutathione, which is intimately involved in immune system health. Glutamine also contributes to growth hormone release and is a key component for intestinal health. For more detailed and referenced information on this remarkable amino acid, please read Dr. Bill Misner's article, "Glutamine Benefits," on the Hammer Nutrition website.

How much do you need?

How much protein do endurance athletes need to consume? Numerous studies have demonstrated that endurance athletes in heavy training need more protein than recreational athletes do. Previously, it was believed that 1/2 gram of protein per pound (about 1/2 kilogram) of body weight—75 grams for a 150-pound (68 kg) person—per day was sufficient. Today's standards, however, would increase that figure to about 100-112 grams (2/3 to 3/4 grams of protein per pound of body weight).

To find out how much you require, multiply your weight in kilograms by 1.4 to 1.7, depending on your exercise intensity. This gives you the amount of protein (in grams) that you should consume on a daily basis. (To convert from pounds to kilograms, divide by 2.2.) Thus, a 165-pound (75 kg) athlete in high training mode should consume about 128 grams of protein daily.

In real-life amounts, to obtain 128 grams of protein you would need to consume a quart of skim milk (32 grams), 3 oz. of tuna (15 grams), 7 oz. of lean chicken breast (62 grams), 4 slices of whole wheat bread (16 grams), and a few bananas (one gram each).

Of course, we get protein in some amounts from a variety of foods. But how many of us down the equivalent of a quart of milk, a half-can of tuna, two chicken breasts, and four slices of whole wheat bread every day? Track and record your diet and do some calculating. It takes quite a bit of effort to ensure adequate protein intake, especially for vegetarians and those who avoid dairy products. Remember to include protein intake from Sustained Energy, Perpetuem, and Recoverite in your calculations. If you still come up short, consider additional applications of Hammer Whey and/or Hammer Soy. If you're serious about your performance and your health, then respect the importance of acquiring adequate protein in your diet.

SUMMARY

Obtaining adequate amounts of protein in the diet is crucial for endurance athletes.

Although it's not given the same kind of "status" as carbohydrates, there is no doubt that obtaining adequate amounts of protein in the diet is crucial for endurance athletes. Use the information in this article to help you determine what kind of protein to use and how much, and start reaping the athletic performance and overall health benefits!

Priceless knowledge is yours for FREE!

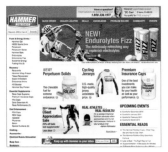

Hammer Nutrition Website

The Hammer Nutrition website has been designed with your needs in mind. Our website offers a user-friendly look and feel with easy access to our entire line of products. Visit our website today for everything from the latest information on our premier products to our unparalleled wealth of knowledge for improving your performance.

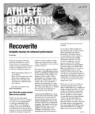

Athlete Education Series

The Athlete Education Series is a printed weekly resource that provides the science and rationale behind specific Hammer Nutrition fuels and supplements, along with other helpful tips. Armed with this information, you'll have a greater knowledge of the various Hammer Nutrition products, what they contain and why, and how best to use them.

FREE electronic subscription
Go to www.hammernutrition.com/AES

Endurance News

Our free magazine, published every 60 days, features insightful articles on diet, nutrition, training, and other topics of interest to endurance athletes, including how to optimize the use of Hammer Nutrition fuels and supplements. More than 84 full-color pages of helpful information. Published continuously since 1992.

FREE electronic subscription
Go to www.hammernutrition.com/EN

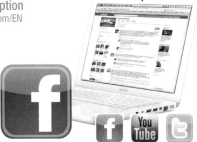

Virtual Community

Like us on Facebook! Check our Facebook wall frequently for up-to-date happenings, including various events that we'll be attending with free samples, new product announcements, product knowledge, special offers, and more. Look for us on Flickr, YouTube, and Twitter too!

Video

Short, instructional videos are the latest addition to our extensive information offerings. Visit the Hammer Nutrition website where you'll be able to watch and listen to Steve Born and Dustin Phillips provide information on each of the Hammer Nutrition products, optimal usage, and our fueling strategies.

Endurance Forum

Our "clients only" discussion group hosted by Brian Frank, Steve Born, and a panel of professional athletes, coaches, and experts in just about anything even remotely related to endurance training. Have all of your questions answered, share ideas, and learn with our friendly community.
www.hammernutrition.com/forums/